Praise for *Preserve Your Brain ...*

"This wonderful resource explains how to optimize your brain, and the science behind it, in easy to understand language and pictures."

Debbie Hampton, Author
The Best Brain Possible
www.thebestbrainpossible.com

"I regularly share many of these simple methods in my classes. Students find them enormously helpful for their clients and themselves, in managing stress and enhancing vitality."

Dr. Rita Marinoble, Professor of Counselor Education
California State University at Sacramento

"If you want more energy, focus and clarity, use this book! You will be amazed. From classrooms to board meetings to therapy groups of all ages, I've used these techniques, and they bring fast results."

Louise Peloquin, Ph.D., Psychotherapist
Fort Myers, Florida

"Vibrant health includes physical and mental stamina to meet the challenges of life. I enjoy these brain-boosting exercises in Ann's classes, for increasing overall fitness."

Pete Kokinda, Middle School Principal
and Physical Education Teacher (Ret.)
Lake County, Indiana

Preserve Your BRAIN

Tools for Growing Mental Fitness

Ann Marina

Please Note:
To reduce the risk of injury, never force or strain during exercise.

Disclaimer:
The information in this book is for educational purposes, and is not intended to serve as medical advice or treatment. If you have any physical or mental health concerns, please consult with a medical or mental health care professional.

The mention of any company, product, or organization does not imply endorsement by the author.

The author disclaims all liability arising directly or indirectly from your use of this book.

ISBN-13: 978-1490973562
ISBN-10: 1490973567

First Edition

For further information, visit: http://www.preserveyourbrain.com

Dedication

To everyone who uses this book.
I hope you'll enjoy and benefit by it.

Acknowledgements

SPECIAL THANKS
"Start-Up Campaign" Contributors
Your support brought this book to life!

Susan Kolanda
Mary Lee Ryan
Viviann Plenge
Jane Kiester
John & Barb Gambles
Rosemary Purdy
Angela Giammarco
Becky Niehoff
Teresa Desilco
Nancy Casey
James Ake
Kitty Johnson
Lynn Gallo

Patty Rubino
Nancy Medis
Martina McNaboe
Carl & Sandy Marchetti
Joan Dugas
Rita Marinoble
Phyllis Mathews
Mary Lou Desco
Peggy Bradley
Eunice & Jeff Cresswell
Linda Baker
Margret Wiens
David & Judy Hall

With Gratitude for your part in the production:

Cindi Ryerson, RN, Director, Millennium Cognitive Café of Southwest Florida, for hosting my first brain fitness class
Richard Evans, for expert photography advice
Angela Giammarco
Erika Cooper
James Ake
Margret Wiens
Mary Lou Desco
   for modeling the exercises in the photos
All persons I've met through yoga, tai chi, and meditation groups, for inspiring me

CONTENTS

Introduction

WE GROW NEW BRAIN CELLS and streamline their connections by engaging our bodies and minds.

When we laugh, sing, take a walk, or learn new things, it builds and improves our brain circuits.

Prior to 1998, conventional science held that when brain cells die, they are not replaced. It was considered normal for human brains to steadily decline with age.

Then at the Salk Institute, Professor Fred Gage published a landmark study confirming neurogenesis, the growth of new cells in human brains. The discovery forced scientists to rethink basic concepts about the brain.

Dr. Gage and his team also showed that physical exercise enhances nerve cell growth in the brain.[1]

Since then, a flurry of research continues to verify our brains' adaptability, known as "neuroplasticity."

"Connections are forged and strengthened between brain areas that work together," writes Robin Brey, M.D., in *Neuorology Now*. The best part is: this happens regardless of one's age.[2]

A study of London cab drivers showed they each had a hippocampus larger than that of subjects who had not learned the map of that city. The cabbies spend at least two years mastering the bewildering maze of streets in London, and take a stringent exam to get the job.

As the hippocampus affects spatial learning and memory, it was no surprise that the amount of growth correlated with how much experience the drivers had. Researchers noted the "capacity for local plastic change in the healthy adult brain in response to environmental demands."[3]

The hippocampus is active as we recall people's names, where we put the car keys, why we entered a room, etc. Keeping it "blooming" with new neurons helps preserve our memory circuits.

The focus of this book is whole brain activation through postures, breathing, and synchronized movements.

Your hippocampus and frontal lobes will sprout new cells with regular practice of the "crossover" moves.[4] And your cerebellum will activate, to improve balance, mental focus, and processing speed.[5]

The exercises draw from yoga, tai chi, coordination movements (described in Chapter 2), meditation, and acupressure.

Although I've practiced these mind-body fitness methods for many years, I only recently learned how they directly benefit the brain.

I'm in the "Baby Boomer" generation, along with many of my class members. We're encouraged by the potentials for enhancing brain vitality as we age.

We have fun with these exercises, and I hope you will, too.

1

Your Brain Circuits

YOU HAVE ABOUT 100 BILLION neurons and a trillion glial cells in your three-pound miracle, the brain.

Neurons, the main working cells of the brain, are supported by the glial cells, which form protective sheaths around them, and take up toxins that may damage them.

Projecting from each neuron is an axon, a long thin structure that carries impulses to other brain cells. A huge axon network in your brain conveys signals to form mental concepts and sensory impulses.

Dendrites also emanate from neurons. They are shorter extensions with branches, resembling trees. Dendrites receive impulses from other neurons at the synapse, a gap where the axon conveys a signal to the dendrite of a neighboring neuron.

In the gap (synapse), electrical signals from the axon change into chemical signals. They are then converted back into electrical signals by neurotransmitter receptors on the receiving neuron's dendrite.

These electrical signals are funneled toward the receiving cell's body. If enough electrical signals arrive together, the signal is passed farther along a chain of neurons.

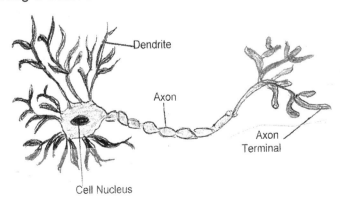

Aging and Brain Reserve

As you age, the number of synaptic connections decreases, notably in the hippocampus and prefrontal cortex. There is shrinking of some neurons and retracting of their dendrites, which can atrophy if their synapses are not being engaged.[1]

In 1979, Stephen Buell and Paul Coleman examined the brains of adults with senile dementia (average age 76) and adults with no signs of dementia (average age 79). They found far less dendrites in the brains of those affected by dementia.[2]

The good news: You add more synapses by exercising and learning new things. Accumulating synapses creates a "brain reserve"—ensuring its continued vitality.

Just as saving money for retirement prepares you for financial challenges later in life, stimulating your brain to form synapses helps you resist adversities such as Alzheimer's, says Majid Fotuhi, M.D. He is chair of the Neurology Institute for Brain Health and Fitness, and assistant professor of neurology at Johns Hopkins University.

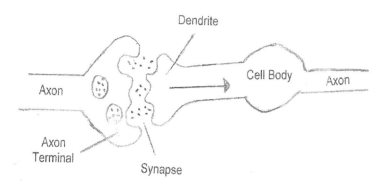

To keep growing synapses, Dr. Fotuhi recommends coordinated movements (like the ones in this book). An avid dancer, he demonstrated the tango with his wife on a PBS TV special, *Fight Alzheimer's Early.*

"Nearly the entire brain becomes active when you dance," he says. "You're using balance, coordination, spatial orientation, and memory all at once."

(*Don't worry,* mastering the tango is not required for a fit brain!)

Sprouting new synapses "makes the brain much richer and denser," adds Dr. Fotuhi.[3]

Rewiring the Circuits

Based on neuroplasticity, there have been exciting advances in rehabilitation for stroke, head injuries, and other brain traumas where patients lose the use of a limb.

In Constraint-Induced Movement Therapy (CIMT), the patient's "good" arm or hand is kept in a sling or a bulky cloth mitt, forcing the use of the affected limb. In the past decade, CIMT has helped many patients gradually restore function in their affected limbs.

Magnetic images of successful CIMT patients' brains reveal new brain circuits that have grown around the damaged wiring as they regain use of their limbs.[4,5]

Lobes of the Brain

There are five main lobes, or regions, in your brain. Each is responsible for a different task:

Frontal and prefrontal—judgment, decisions, taking actions.

Temporal—memory and mood stability.

Parietal—sensory processing and sense of direction.

Occipital—visual information processing.

Cerebellum—movement and coordination.

Back and Front Halves

In general, the back half of your brain is receptive and perceptive, while the front half carries out "executive functions"—making decisions and directing actions.

These receptive and expressive functions are summarized by Dr. Daniel Amen in *Magnificent Mind At Any Age:*

The back half of your brain—the parietal, occipital, and back of the temporal lobes—takes in and perceives the world. The front half integrates the information, decides what to do, then plans and executes the action.[6]

Left and Right Hemispheres

The left hemisphere is active when you use the right side of your body. The right hemisphere is active for the left side of your body.[7]

The left side tends to focus on details, analysis and logic; it likes mathematics. The right side is involved with music and art, seeing "the big picture", intuition and creativity. In some people, however, these functions are transposed.[8]

Where Memories Live

A single memory is not stored in just one place in your brain. For example, your memory of an apple consists of how it looks, tastes, the crunchy sound, etc. Information about the apple is stored in different places in your brain, which must be accessed for you to recall an apple.

Dr. Aaron Nelson describes the process in The Harvard Medical School Guide to Achieving Optimal Memory:

"Its visual form is stored in the occipital lobe. How it tastes is stored in the gustatory cortex in the insula and the amygdala. The sound of its crunch is in the temporal lobes, and its name is stored in the left temporal and parietal lobes," he writes.

"... to retrieve your memory of an apple, all of these brain regions become activated and work in concert to recombine the 'experience' of apple into a complete whole, like instruments in an orchestra playing together to create a symphony." [9]

Nourishing Your Brain

Here's more good news for preserving your brain. Neurons have nerve growth factors—protein molecules called neurotrophins—which keep them healthy and growing. They only flourish in *active* neurons.

Exercising enhances the growth factor BDNF (Brain Derived Neurotrophic Factor). John Ratey, M.D., praises BDNF as "miracle-gro for the brain" in *Spark, the Revolutionary New Science of Exercise and the Brain.* [10]

Studies have shown that BDNF levels are lower in Alzheimer's patients. BDNF improves connections between neurons and aids in forming new synapses, vital for thinking, and learning, writes David Perlmutter, M.D., in *Power Up Your Brain.*[11]

Neurons must be sending or receiving signals, to respond well to neurotrophins. The more active a neuron is, the more growth factors it produces, and the better it can use those it receives from other neurons.[12]

Regular physical activity ensures that your brain is well-nourished.

2

How The Exercises Work

YOUR BRAIN'S HUNDRED BILLION neurons communicate through an estimated quadrillion connections. Thus, the possible combination of nerve messages traveling in a brain exceeds the number of known atoms in the universe! [1]

Every thought or experience makes a neural connection. If you repeat that thought or experience, the connection grows stronger, paving a "circuit", or energy pathway.

"Neurons that fire together, wire together" is a popular phrase describing the concept first proposed by Sigmund Freud: neurons form electrical communication lines based on simultaneous firings.

"With repetition, you create thicker myelin around the nerve fibers, which improves the quality and speed of the signals, and in turn, the circuit's efficiency," observes John Ratey, M.D., in *SPARK: The Revolutionary New Science of Exercise and the Brain.*[2]

Brains physically change as we exercise, learn skills and store information. Thus, when you go to a class or hit the gym, you return with a different brain. Really.

Like improving a road system, the exercises in this book streamline your brain's circuits, to enhance memory, clarity, and sense of balance. They activate your whole brain by working various parts of it in unison.

Attention Is Key

Your brain loves activities requiring highly focused attention. In *The Brain That Changes Itself,* Dr. Norman Doidge explains that the more attentively we focus, the better our brains participate in an activity and benefit from it.

When you are attentive, your brain produces chemicals such as dopamine, a neurotransmitter which keeps your energy and motivation rolling.[3]

The tools in this book engage your attention by challenging your balance and concentration skills.

Coordination Movements

Repeated crossing of your body's midline with arms or legs, like touching your left knee with right hand, then right knee with left hand, synchronizes the two brain hemispheres.

This involves the corpus callosum, a bundle of nerve fibers connecting left and right sides of your brain. It is active in problem solving and creativity.

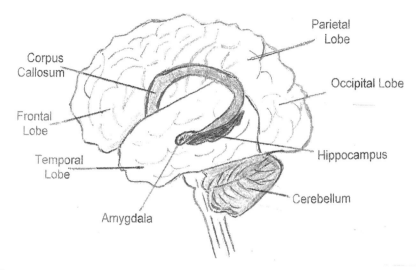

Crossovers speed up communication between hemispheres, for integration and high-level reasoning, explains Carla Hannaford, Ph.D., in *Smart Moves.*[4]

"A coordinated series of movements, done slowly with balance, produces increased neurotrophins (nerve growth factors), more connections among neurons, and nerve cell growth, especially in the hippocampus and frontal lobes of the brain," Hannaford adds.[5]

Coordinated movements are also done without crossing midline. In tai chi, we step forward with the left foot while punching with the right fist. Many moves and postures in tai chi engage all our limbs at once, and the continual weight shifting requires full attention, to avoid toppling over!

A few exercises in this toolkit are from tai chi movements.

Your Cerebellum

As you coordinate movements, the cerebellum gets involved. Located at the back bottom of your brain, it's about the size of a plum and contains nearly half of all the brain's neurons! The cerebellum affects balance and motor activities, and the processing of thoughts and information.

Engaging the cerebellum helps you think faster and more clearly. It improves judgment, attention and overall brain health, writes Dr. Daniel Amen, in *Making A Good Brain Great*.[6]

Whole-Brain Activation

With your hands, feet and eyes involved in the crossover moves, you're calling on various brain regions to work together, including the front and back brains. It causes your brain's receptive and expressive areas to work in harmony, assisting with learning, focus, and memory skills.

When babies first begin crawling, their corpus callosum is activated by the cross-lateral movements. With both sides of the body and brain working together, the child's actions become more integrated. Educators have known for decades that the crawling stage is essential in developing good learning and thinking skills.

The popular Brain Gym® program uses coordination and other exercises involving both the expressive and receptive sides of the brain. Since the 1970s, Brain Gym® has been helping children and adults to focus in academics or sports, often with amazingly fast improvements.[7]

You may have seen Dr. Daniel Amen on PBS TV's *Use Your Brain To Change Your Age*. Dr. Amen recommends Brain Gym® and the Interactive Metronome program (IM) for better coordination and cognitive processing. Participants in the IM program work to synchronize hand and foot movements to a rhythmic beat generated by a computer.[8,9]

Besides coordination movements, this book presents breathing, balancing postures, eye and hand movements, meditation, laughing and smiling. *Yes, laughing and smiling* are natural brain-builders. You probably already knew that.

Brain Gym® is a registered trademark of Brain Gym® International/ Educational Kinesiology Foundation

Your concentration will be challenged in some of these, such as drawing 8's with one hand while you draw 0's with the other.

Your overall health will benefit by the stretching, twisting, breathing, and laughing.

Whether you're in top athletic shape, or have limited mobility, you can do most of the exercises in this book. Suggestions for adaptations are provided.

Movement is essential for preserving a healthy brain. "Exercise promotes the production of new cells in the hippocampus," notes Jorg Blech in *Healing Through Exercise*. "It also creates new synapses, for establishing and maintaining the vast network of connected nerve cells in the brain." [10]

3

Using This Book

THIS TOOLKIT IS LOADED WITH many effective techniques, and I do not expect you to use them all at once!

Browse through the exercises and lifestyle tips. Find out what sparks your interest, and get going. Have fun.

Choose your exercises

You know best what your brain needs. Sometimes 30 seconds of conscious breathing will refresh your mind, or a 3-minute set can help you focus. At other times, you may want longer routines. Use the "Brain workout charts" in Chapter 6 to make your own sets.

Know Your Goals, Build Your Workouts

Check out the sample sets, such as "1-Minute Refresher" and "5-Minute Brain Builder". You can use these for your workouts, and/or choose from the Summary to build your own sets.

The exercises are grouped under Activators (energizers) or Refreshers (the more calming ones) in Chapter 6, the Summary.

Don't worry about categories... just go with the exercises that feel good and suit your needs.

In general:

Activators help "switch your brain on" for energy, clarity, better memory and concentration.

Refreshers are great for balance, calming and stress relief.

Vary the Exercises

You can substitute exercises shown in the sample sets, with similar ones from the Summary, i.e., replace one crossover with another. A few exercises appear in more than one set, due to their types of benefits.

Move Slowly Across Midline

This requires more fine motor involvement and balance, which activates your vestibular system and strengthens signaling between hemispheres.[1]

Enjoy a physical workout
Most exercises encourage a good stretch or twist.

Link your breathing with movements
This helps you stay "present" in your body and creates a rhythm, for full brain activation. For example, inhaling as arms go up, exhaling as they go down. You'll see reminders in the instructions.

Drink Water! It conducts electricity, and keeps your energy flowing.

Clothing and Yoga Mat
All you need are bare feet or comfortable, supportive shoes, and clothing suitable for stretching. And your smile! ☺ I recommend using a yoga mat to prevent slipping. They are reasonably priced at sporting goods stores and many large department stores.

When To Practice
Any time! If you need a boost, or a moment's refuge on a hectic day, one or two exercises can help, *or -*
Include a set in your regular daily workout, *or -*
Perhaps in the morning, with your coffee, tea, or green smoothie?

How Long; How Often?
For serious brain building, take at least 10 minutes a day, 5 days a week. If you're already doing regular physical and mental workouts, just a few times a week will suffice, to supplement your routine.

As You Begin
Read instructions, look at photos, and practice things that are new to you. Soon you'll have your favorite exercises memorized.

"Stretch, don't strain" is our motto. No forcing of movements. Many can be done seated, or holding a solid support like a counter top, table, or wall.

Resources and References
See Endnotes for reference citations. The Resources section has sources of brain fitness information—just the tip of the iceberg!

Brain Builder's Terms

You will encounter these along the way.

Adaptation

Optional ways to perform an exercise, i.e., "Can be done while seated," or "Hold a sturdy support as you balance on one leg."

Breathing – is mentioned often in the exercises. Breathe normally, except in specific Deep Breathing techniques.

Cognitive Skills

Intellectual activity such as thinking, reasoning, recalling facts, and making decisions.

Consideration

gives a precaution about an exercise.

Corpus Callosum

A bundle of nerve fibers connecting left and right brain hemispheres. Nerve messages travel back and forth across it in the coordination exercises. Energy circuits form and grow stronger in the corpus callosum with regular practice of crossover movements. This streamlines the communication between your two brain hemispheres.[2]

Crossover: Your arm or leg is reaching across your body's midline.

Full brain activation

This occurs when large areas of both hemispheres are engaged.

Hip-width or Shoulder-Width apart *(referring to your feet)*

The *outer edges* of your feet are basically in line with outer edges of shoulders or hips. Check the spacing of your feet for good stability.

Holding a posture

It takes time for the experience of a posture to "sink in". I usually recommend holding for at least 5 breaths, as do many yoga teachers.

Your brain gets busy while you're holding a posture! It checks to make sure you're balanced, and not toppling over. It communicates with muscles as they're stretching, so they don't tear.

Holding a stretch helps you become more flexible, so you can stretch farther with practice.

Mindfulness is maintaining awareness of thoughts and sensations.

Nerve messaging

Communication between brain cells, as you move or hold a stretch. The exercises in this book can help increase your brain's nerve growth hormone, through repetition of nerve messaging.

Repetition

...gets the pattern established in your brain as neurons create and strengthen their pathways of communication.

Smile as you exercise?

Yes! It releases endorphins in your brain to increase energy and enthusiasm.[3]

Tongue Tip Resting on Roof of Mouth

It's not required, but you may want to try this Kinesiology method. It enhances focus and balance by stimulating tongue ligaments connecting to the vestibular system.[4] It also helps your jaw relax. Some people keep the tongue tip there while exercising.

Try resting it comfortably on the palate just behind your upper teeth, or more toward the center of your palate.

4

Sample Exercises

Bear Walk, Human Walk ...a primer

Benefit: You'll notice the natural movements of your limbs as you walk. "Contralateral" arm and leg movements engage both sides of the brain when you walk naturally. Coordinated contralateral moves are used in many brain-building exercises.

Actions: Pretend you're a big bear, lumbering along with shoulders hunched forward. As you walk, bring the same side arm forward with each foot. Right arm goes forward with right foot, and left arm with left foot. This is homo-lateral movement. After taking several steps this way, straighten up and walk normally. Notice how your opposite arm naturally comes forward with each foot, in the contra-lateral way humans walk.

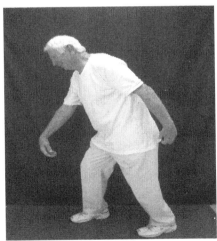
Bear Walk

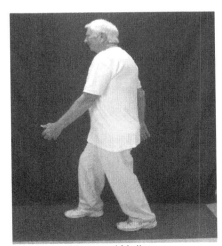
Human Walk

Four Basic Exercises

To get a feel for brain building activities. Enjoy!

Beach Ball Twist

Benefits: Crossing midline stimulates nerve messages between brain hemispheres, so your receptive and expressive sides work together. Challenges your balance and tones the abdominals.

Actions: Imagine holding a beach ball at your right hip. Lift your right knee across your midline and point it to the left front corner. Optional: touch your right hip with left hand as you go. Come back to center, and repeat on the other side. Go back and forth, tossing 8 times to each side.

BREATHE with the movements, exhaling on each toss.

Adaptations: You could hold a sturdy support with one hand, while "tossing back" with the other.

If lifting your knee is a problem, cross one straight leg in front of the other, and tap the toe down in front.

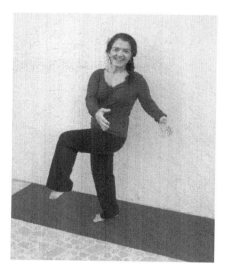 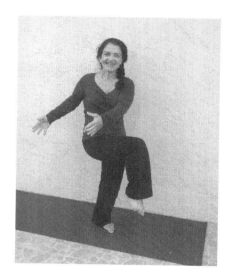

Put your love to work to help heal the planet. You are important.
Louise Hay

V for Vitality

Opens the lungs for enhanced breathing. Crossing your arms stimulates messaging across the corpus callosum.

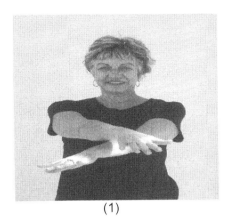

(1)

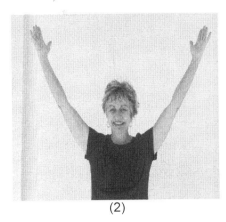

(2)

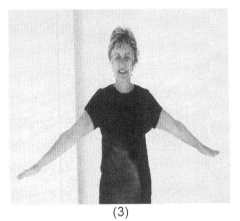

(3)

Actions: Stand with feet shoulder-width apart. Raise both arms out in front of you. Cross forearms, and then lift and separate them, like a "V". Breathe in as you lift and open; Breathe out as you bring arms down by your sides.

Repeat, alternating the arm on top, for a total of 8 circles.

Adaptation: May be done in a chair. If your shoulders feel strained, try lifting your arms just halfway up.

Trace the Wheel

Benefits: Improves alertness and concentration. Makes you laugh or smile, I hope. Synchronizes left and right hemispheres.
Actions: Can be done seated, or standing with one foot a half step in front and knees slightly bent, for stability.

(1) With your right hand, reach out, as if to shake someone's hand. Now imagine "tracing a wheel" in this way: your fingers point UP as they come in toward your chest, then DOWN as your hand moves outward, along the "wheel edge". Repeat the circling motion 3 more times. That's easy.
(2) Now draw the wheel with your *Left hand only*...but the fingers go the *opposite way*. Left fingers point UP as they move <u>away</u> from you, and DOWN as they draw in toward you, to complete the circle. Practice circling the Left hand in this direction several times.
(3) *Your CHALLENGE:* Draw the wheel with both hands at once. Your fingers move in opposite directions: Right fingers point UP as they come IN towards your chest; and Left fingers point UP as they move OUT.

The more we do it, the easier it gets.

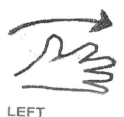

LEFT

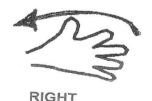

RIGHT

Mindful Breathing

Benefits: Brings calm and focus to a chattering mind. Award-winning actress and author of *10 Mindful Minutes,* Goldie Hawn wrote, "Mindful breathing helps create a balanced neurosystem, for healthy brain function.

Mindfulness is the conscious awareness of our current thoughts, feelings, and surroundings, and accepting this awareness...in a non-judgmental way. It means focusing our attention on *nondoing*, a crucial skill in these distracted times." [1]

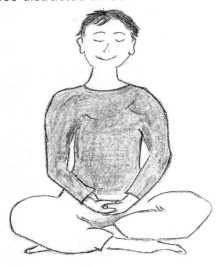

Action: Sitting comfortably (or lying down), feel the breath flowing in and out of your nostrils. Feel your ribcage expand on each inhale, and your whole body releasing with each exhale. Notice the pause – a moment of calm stillness - after each exhale, just before the next inhale. Relax and enjoy mindful breathing for about one minute.

Options: (1) Keep a slight smile going in this exercise, to increase your brain benefits. (2) With eyes closed, look up toward your brow-point (known as the "3rd eye") on your forehead, midway between the eyebrows and a half-inch or so above. Doing this helps some people focus in meditation. *It takes some practice before it feels comfortable.*

5

Exercise Sets

THESE ARE SAMPLE SETS of varying lengths, containing just a portion of all the exercises. Some are in more than one set, due to their particular benefits.

If the first sets seem boring, zip down to "Challengers" – that's the last set.

The Exercise Summary in Chapter 6 lists all the exercises, grouped by their primary benefits.

Feel the beat!
To keep your energy humming, you could put on some favorite tunes, and move in time with the beat.

Timing the exercises?
Use a clock or watch that shows the seconds (if you're concerned about time) or just use your intuition. ☺ Stated times are flexible.

Drink water. Breathe.
Before starting, take a few conscious breaths and sips of water, for focused attention and good circulation.

Smile.
For even more brain benefits.

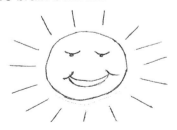

5-Minute Brain Builder

This set has coordinated movements for whole-brain activation. Your expressive and receptive hemispheres are working in unison.

8's in the Sky

Benefits: Activates left and right hemispheres in unison; limbers the shoulders and enhances your breathing.

Actions: Stand with your knees slightly bent and feet shoulder-width apart, for a solid stance. Raise your right arm straight out in front of you, at chest height. Draw a big sideways figure 8 in the air with your right hand. Or you could draw it on a large chalk board.

As you move, let your weight shift a little, from side to side.

Draw it 5 times with your right hand, and then 5 times with your left. Now draw it 5 times with both hands, one resting on the other.

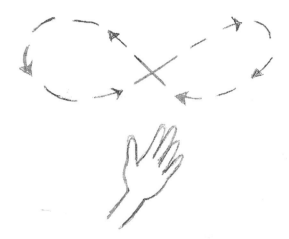

Tips:

(1) Draw upward through the center of the "8", as Dr. Hannaford suggests, to follow the energy through your midline.

(2) Focus on the "X" at center of the 8 to engage neural pathways of the corpus callosum, and synchronize your brain hemispheres.[1]

(3) Make the 8 wider than your shoulders and higher than your head, to really work your arms and get brain hemispheres engaged.

8's and 0's = A Challenge!

Benefits: Aids concentration. Makes you laugh or smile (I hope). Connects the two cerebral hemispheres.

Actions: As in 8's in the Sky, you're standing with feet shoulder-width apart. Raise your right arm to chest height. Draw a sideways figure 8 in the air with your right hand. Do this a few times, and then,
> ***Your challenge:***
> Draw a circle in the air with your left hand, while you draw the 8 with your right hand. Draw at least 4, and then change sides: do a circle with your right hand, and sideways 8 with your left. Interesting? Repeat the sequence at least once more.

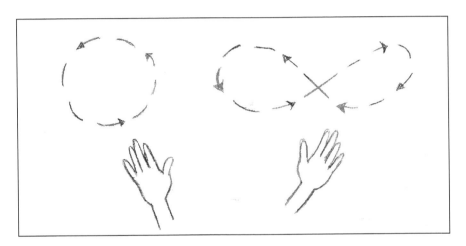

A Tougher Challenge ...

8's and 0's with Feet!
Lying on your back, or sitting with your back supported, lift your legs and do the same figures with your feet, instead of your hands. *Fun!*
Bend your knees, if it feels better for your back.

Same - Same

*I recommend this unique exercise **only if** your energy is very low,* and the crossovers feel like a struggle. And/or do the "Bear Walk" in Chapter 4. To help you get moving, do them **before** crossovers.

Our energies normally "criss-cross" over the body's midline, as the right brain controls the left side of the body, and vice versa.

At times, however, we feel sluggish—our energy gets "stuck." It moves weakly up and down each side, without crossing center.

Do you ever feel "mentally foggy", first thing in the morning, or after sitting at the computer for hours? It may also occur after an illness or a long period of inactivity.[2,3]

Benefit: Gets your energy moving along homo-lateral lines, on either side of the body. Once it's moving well, it's easier to make the crossover moves!

Actions: Standing with feet about hip-width apart, inhale and lift your left arm and left knee at the same time. As you exhale, lower the left arm and leg, and lift your right arm and leg. Go back and forth, slowly, for at least 8 lifts *on each side.* NOW you're ready for the Activator Exercises.

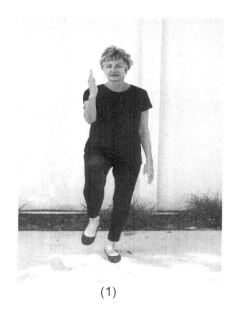

(1)

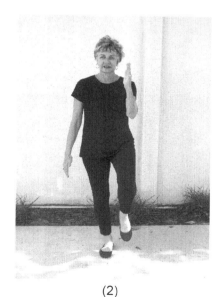

(2)

Crossover
(or try a Crossover Challenge on next page)

Benefit: Crossing midline in a rhythmic pattern activates the two hemispheres in unison. The brain "switches on" with these moves.

Actions: Stand with your feet about hip-width apart. Reach your left hand across to touch the right knee as you raise it, and then do the same with the right hand on the left knee. As if slowly "marching in place", continue for 30 seconds or more.

Adaptation: Can be done while seated.

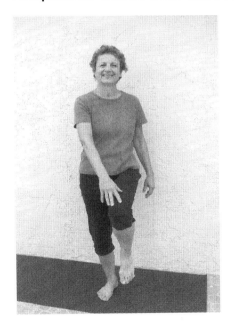 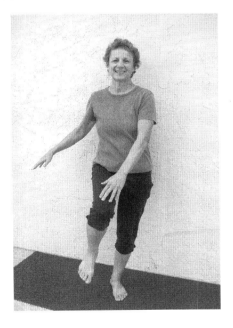

"A balanced brain is the foundation for a life that is happier, healthier, wealthier, and wiser."
- Daniel Amen, M.D.

Crossover Challenges

These challenge your balance and give you more of a twist. *Try one or more, without forcing any stretches.*

Benefits: Full brain activation by crossing your midline.

Actions:

Go at least 30 seconds, side to side, coordinating your breath with the movements:

(1) Cross over and touch right elbow to left knee, and then left elbow to right knee.

(2) Lift your foot and cross over to touch it. 3) Kick a foot up behind you. Reach behind with opposite side hand to touch it.

Adaptations: #1 and 2 can be done while seated. #3 could be done with a counter top or other sturdy support in front of you. Place one hand on the support.

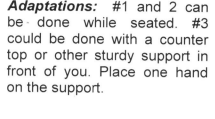

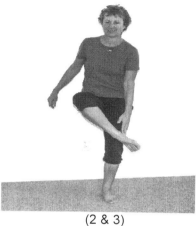

(2 & 3)

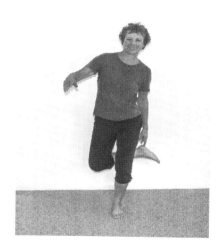

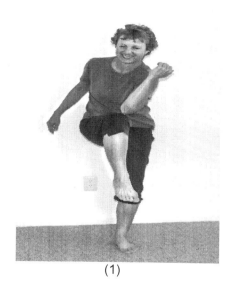

(1)

Swingin' *(Easier than crossovers)*

Benefit: Both arms cross your midline at once, for whole brain activation. The twisting burns calories and trims your waistline.

Actions: With knees bent and feet about shoulder-width apart, enjoy swinging your arms. Let your hips sway, and weight shift side to side. As the arms cross your midline, touch left hip with right hand, and if possible, bring your left hand around behind you to touch the right hip. Keep swingin' arms back and forth across midline, and tapping hips.
Breathe! Keep your shoulders relaxed, and go at least 30 seconds.

Adaptation: The arm movements can be done while seated.

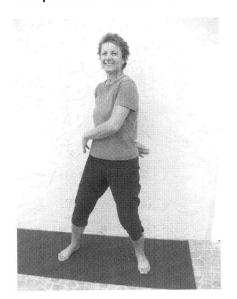 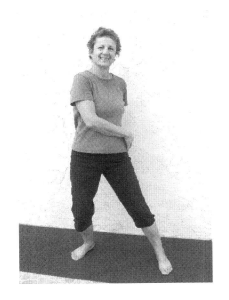

"Exercise cues the building blocks
of learning in the brain."
John Ratey, M.D.

Seated Side Stretch

Benefits:

Crossing midline provides full brain activation. This stretch relieves tension in hips and back, opens the lungs and increases your energy with improved circulation.

Actions:

Sitting up tall, with right hand on your left thigh.

Keep the hip down on your left side, and reach your left arm over your head toward the right wall. Relax into the stretch and breathe.

Think of the letter "C" (as your raised arm is in that shape, and you're keeping it above your head).

Hold for a few breaths, and then change sides. Repeat once more on each side.

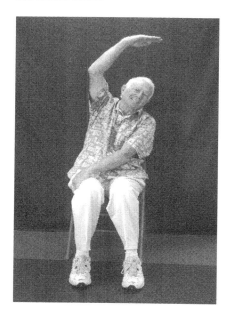 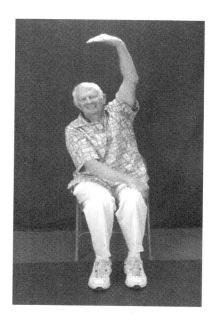

A person's mind, once stretched by a new idea, never regains its original dimension. –Oliver Wendell Holmes

Columns

Benefit: "Switches the brain on" for energy and mental clarity, as nerve messages travel between the two hemispheres. Research at Manchester University in England found that moving eyes horizontally, back and forth, may improve short-term memory skills.[4]

Actions: With eyes closed, picture two vertical columns. The left one has letters going down it: A,B,C,D, and E. The right column has numbers going down, from 1 through 5. Visualize enough space between your columns so your eyes must move side to side in this exercise.

> *Smile;* keep your eyes closed.
> Look back and forth from left to right, as you count.
> A-1, B-2, etc... to E-5.
>
> Now reverse direction, from right to left.
> 1-A, 2-B ... to 5-E.
> Rest your eyes for a few breaths, and repeat this exercise at least once more.

A -- 1

B -- 2

C -- 3

D -- 4

E -- 5

Deep Breathing

This is a three-part breath. You can take in seven times as much oxygen in this breath than in a shallow breath, says Integral Yoga Instructor Swami Karunananda.[5]

Benefits: Energizes you with fresh oxygen reaching the brain and vital organs through your bloodstream.

Actions: *Lie on your back* with knees bent and feet flat on the floor (or bed), hip-width apart. Picture your abdomen and chest as a balloon filling from the bottom up as you inhale.

First your abdomen expands, then the rib cage, and third is the upper chest. On your exhale, it follows the same order: first the abdomen sinks back down, then the rib cage and the chest. Finally, pull your abdomen in slightly to empty the lungs completely.

Beginners: try it slowly two or three times, and then rest before doing a few more. If you feel dizzy, stop and rest before you get up.

Experienced breathers may take 5 or 6 breaths; rest and repeat.

Adaptations: May be done in a chair, but you'll feel more rising and falling, and have less possibility of dizziness while lying down.

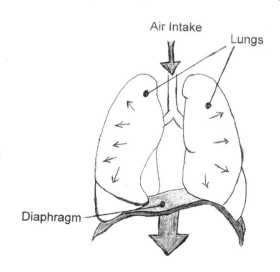

3-Part Inhale: Diaphragm moves down as lungs expand

3-minute Recharge

Standing Forward Bend

Benefits: Calms the brain; helps relieve stress, mild depression, headache and insomnia, according to Yoga Journal. [6]

Precaution: If you feel too much pressure in your eyes or head, do not stay in the forward fold; slowly return to standing.

Actions: Standing up tall, bend forward from the hip joints (from the crease at the top of your legs. This keeps your spine straighter and torso longer than if you curl forward from the waist.) Let your arms dangle, or cross forearms and hold your elbows. Let your head hang from the root of the neck, which is between the shoulder blades. If it feels OK, work your neck a little: gently turn your head side to side or in a circle 2 or 3 times. Hold the position for 20 to 30 seconds. Then bring your hands onto your hips and SLOWLY straighten up.

Adaptations: Rest hands just above your knees while in forward bend. May also be done while seated.

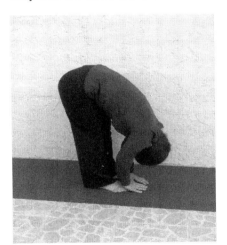 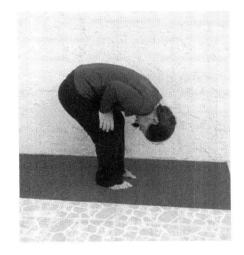

Cow & Cat

Benefits: Enhances energy, metabolism and a positive mood, as tucking chin toward chest stimulates your thyroid gland. More blood reaches the brain through this exercise. Cow and Cat works all the spinal muscles; it increases circulation and relieves tension in your back and neck.

Actions: Start in tabletop position: hands just below shoulders and knees below your hips. Round your spine upward for Cat Pose (like a frightened cat). Tuck your chin gently toward your chest. (Photo 1) Hold for two breaths, then slowly sink your spine downward for cow pose. (Photo 2) You may want to lift your chin and sit bones for more curve in the spine. Do not force the stretch. Hold this for two breaths, then go back and forth at your own pace, inhaling in cow pose and exhaling in cat pose.

Adaptation: May be done seated in a chair, or cross-legged on the floor, curving your spine forward for "cow" and back for "cat". Lifting and lowering your chin is optional.

Share it with the kids! Smile and enjoy.

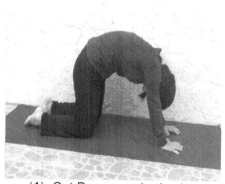
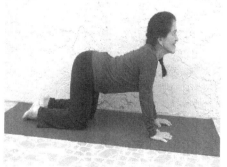

(1) Cat Pose – arched spine with chin tucked.

(2) Cow pose – sunken spine

Downward Dog Pose

Using a yoga mat will prevent your hands and feet from slipping.
In this classic yoga pose, your head is below your heart, so more blood reaches the brain.

Benefits: Calms the nervous system. Relieves tension in neck, shoulders and spinal column. Stretches hamstrings, calves, and arms for energy, circulation, and muscle tone.

Stretching your calf muscles aids the ability to follow through and complete projects, according to Brain Gym®.[7]

Actions: On hands and knees with your hands slightly forward of your shoulders, turn your toes under and lift your hips up high; reach your heels toward the floor, but they don't have to touch it. Press your chest back toward your thighs, so you have a long, straight spine. Relax neck and shoulders, with your head between your upper arms.

Stay in dog pose for several breaths. Rest and repeat.

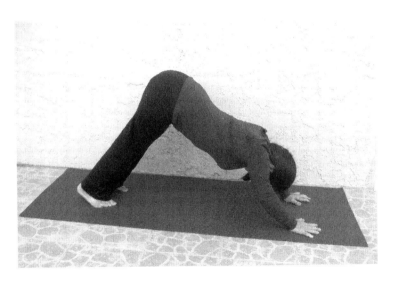

Downward Dog Pose. Relax shoulders and smile!

Seated Twist

Benefits: Crossing midline activates brain hemispheres in unison. Twisting relieves spinal tension and refreshes organs / glands.

Actions: Sitting up tall, place your left hand on your right knee. Turn and look to the left; breathe normally, and with each exhale, relax into the twist. Hold for 3 breaths.
Change sides and repeat, then do 1 more on each side.

Adaptation: For more twist (and brain benefit) cross left knee over the right knee before turning to your left, and cross right knee over left knee, before turning right.

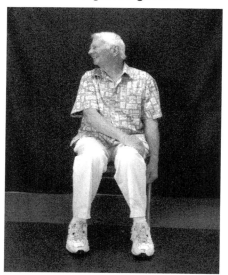

Exhale!
Breathe only as deeply as is comfortable, to avoid dizziness.

Benefits: A deep, "complete" exhale removes old, stale air trapped in your lungs. Energizes you, as your lungs receive fresh, clean air.
Action: *Lying on your back*, inhale deeply. Now purse your lips like you're whistling and slowly blow all the air out, sinking your belly down toward your spine. Even when you think all the air is gone, try to push out a little more. Then feel the clean, refreshing air filling your lungs on the next inhale.

Practice the full exhale at least twice. Then relax with normal breathing a while, before sitting or standing up.

If you get light-headed, stop and rest, lying down and breathing normally for a few minutes. You may want to try it another time.

30-second Zingers
Boost your brain in half a minute! Or go longer, if you wish.

Thumb and Pinky

Benefits: Full brain activation; makes you concentrate and smile!
Actions: Hold your two fists up at about chest-height. Raise just your right thumb and left pinky finger. Then go back to fists. Raise just left thumb and right pinky, and then alternate, several times.
    Too easy? Try speeding up.

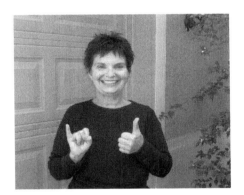 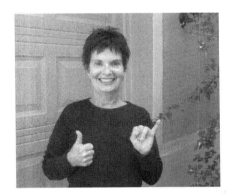

Drawing 8's with eyes

Benefits: "Switches the brain on" for energy and mental clarity, as nerve messages travel between hemispheres. Refreshes tired eyes.
Actions: While seated or lying down, *keep your eyes closed* and draw sideways figure 8's (the infinity symbol) with your eyes. Noticing the X in the center of the 8 will bring more benefits, according to Dr. Hannaford.[8]

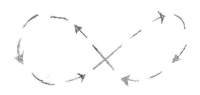

Draw them 4 or 5 times, and then rest for a few breaths. *Smile.*

1-minute Refresher

The Thinking Cap®

This gets "head-turning" results in my classes! (Pun intended.)

Several brain benefits are gained in this exercise. Cecilia Koester, M.Ed., says 98% of those who try it report marked improvement in how far they can turn their heads.[9]

In Traditional Chinese Medicine, acupuncture points on the ears are noted for connecting large nerves to the brain.[10] The Thinking Cap helps relax tension in the neck and bring attention to the auditory system.[11]

One of my class members uses this before playing golf or backing up his car. He says he gets about 20% more head "turn-ability".

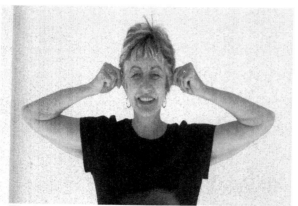

Actions: First, turn your head to the left and see how far you can look without straining your neck. Set a visual marker, like a doorknob. This is how far to the left you can look. Do the same on the right side, setting your visual marker.

Use your thumbs and index fingers to pull your ears gently back and unroll them. Begin at the top of the ear and massage down and around the curve, ending with the bottom lobe. Repeat 3 or more times.

Now, turn your head to the left and notice how far you can look. Is it past your marker? Then turn and check the right marker.

I hope you find it effective.

2-Minute Refresher

Deep Breathing

Three-part breathing is the foundation of all yoga breathing techniques. You can take in seven times as much oxygen in this breath than in a shallow breath, says Integral Yoga Instructor Swami Karunananda.[12]

Benefits: Energizes you with fresh oxygen reaching the brain and vital organs through your bloodstream.

Actions: *Lie on your back* with knees bent and feet flat on the floor (or bed), hip-width apart. Picture your abdomen and chest as a balloon, filling from the bottom up as you inhale.

First your abdomen expands, then the rib cage, and third, the upper chest. On your exhale, it follows the same order: first the abdomen sinks back down, then the rib cage and the chest. Finally, pull your abdomen in again to empty the lungs completely.

Beginners: try it slowly two or three times, and then rest before doing a few more. If you feel dizzy, stop and rest before getting up.

Experienced breathers may take 5 or 6 breaths; rest and repeat.

Adaptations: May be done in a chair, but you'll feel more rising and falling, and have less possibility of dizziness while lying down.

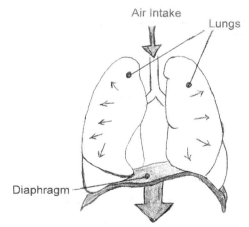

3-part inhale: Diaphragm moves downward as lungs expand

1-Minute Mind Menders

Child Pose

A gentler version can be done in a chair. See "Seated Child Pose" below. Try both arm positions shown. One stretches the muscles along your spine, the other opens the shoulder blade area and relaxes your back.

Benefits: Calms the brain; relieves stress and fatigue. Relaxes your back muscles and stretches hips, thighs and torso.

Actions: Kneel on the floor or mat. Touch your big toes together and sit back by your heels. Separate your knees as wide apart as your hips. Rest your torso down between your thighs. Feel your ribcage expand and contract as you breathe. Relax in the pose for as long as you like.

Variations: (Photo 1) Rest your arms alongside you, palms up, and let your shoulders sink in front of the knees, if they will. Feel the shoulder blades widen across your back. You may prefer (Photo 2) reaching your arms out in front of you, palms down.

Adaptations: If you dislike sitting back by your heels, place a folded blanket between your back thighs and calves.

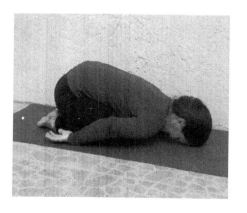 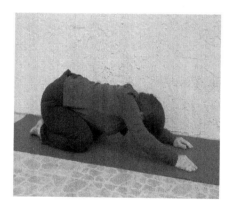

Seated Child Pose

No photo for this. Sitting at a table or desk, place one hand on top of the other, palms down, on the table in front of your chest. Rest your forehead there for a few slow, deep breaths. Then breathe normally with awareness for at least 30 seconds more.

"Energy Link"

I'm sitting on the floor in this photo. You might prefer sitting in a chair or lying on your back.

Benefits: There's a calming effect as you activate the vestibular system to increase focus and balance.

Action: While seated or lying down, cross your ankles and make a pyramid shape with your hands. The pads of fingers and thumbs are touching together. Rest the tip of your tongue on the roof of your mouth, relax and breathe deeply a few times. Now return to normal breathing, holding the posture for at least 30 seconds more.

Adaptations: For a more powerful "energy linking" pose, try the next one, called "Hook-Up."

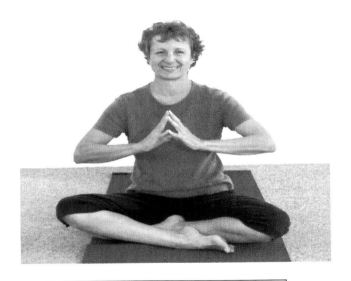

> "Create a solid center for the mind, from which you can act and speak with a good foundation."
> - Thanissaro Bikkhu

Hook-Ups®

Benefits: This Brain Gym® posture invites calm while focusing and organizing scattered attention.[13] It brings attention to the motor cortex of your frontal hemispheres and away from the survival center in the back brain, thus decreasing adrenalin.[14]

Actions: Sitting with your back supported, or lying on your back:

Cross your ankles. It doesn't matter which is on top.

Extend your arms in front of you and cross one wrist over the other.

Interlace your fingers and draw your clasped hands up toward your chest.

Hold like this for a minute or more, breathing slowly, with your eyes open or closed. As you inhale, touch the tip of your tongue to the roof of your mouth at the hard palate (just behind the teeth) and relax your tongue on exhalation.

> **Part Two** *(NOT pictured)*: When ready, uncross your arms and legs and put your fingertips together in front of your chest, continuing to breathe deeply for another minute, and hold the tip of your tongue on the roof of your mouth when you inhale.

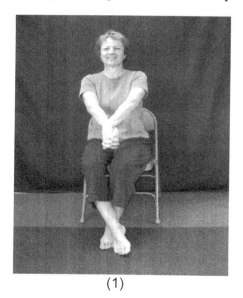

(1)

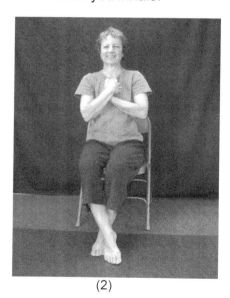

(2)

Pressure Points:

GB 20, *Gates of Consciousness*

Benefits: Regulates circulation to the brain and relaxes the nervous system. Pressing these points helps relieve a stiff neck, insomnia, headache and fatigue. It releases endorphins, the body's natural pain-killers, notes Michael Reed Gach, author, *Acupressure's Potent Points.*[15]

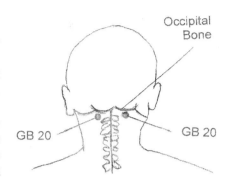

Location: In the hollows just under the base of the skull, on either side of your cervical spine.

Actions: Take a few deep breaths, as you press into these hollows, which are about three inches apart. Tilt your head back slowly and use your thumbs, fingers, or knuckles to gradually apply steady pressure. Hold for one to two minutes, relaxing and breathing with awareness.

K-27, end points of the kidney meridians.

Benefits: Increases the flow of blood to your brain and gets your energy moving, so you feel more alert and positive.[16]

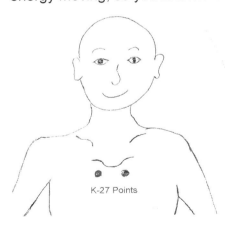

K-27 Points

Location: Just under the collarbone. Place your fingertips on the U-shaped notch at the top of the breastbone, about where a man knots his tie. Then move them out and down about an inch, small depressions there.

Actions: Tap or hold steady pressure on the K-27 points with your two index fingers. Or just use one hand, touching the points with thumb and forefinger. Take a few deep breaths as you tap or hold the points.

Rest for 30 seconds or more.

Alternate Nostril Breath

We use this calming, brain-balancing technique in Yoga class.

Everyone has a "nasal cycle" of air flowing predominantly through one nostril for about one to three hours, and then switching to the other side, according to the National Institutes of Health.[17]

Benefits: Synchronizes the two brain hemispheres. Lowers the heart rate; reduces stress and anxiety.[18,19]

Before starting: Read all the actions, and the note under pictures.

Actions: Sitting with a tall spine, use the *right thumb and ring finger* to gently close off one nostril at a time. Curl your right index and middle finger down into your palm, so just the ring and pinky fingers are up.

Press your ring finger over your left nostril and inhale for 4 counts through your right nostril (Image #1). Close your right nostril with your thumb, so both are now closed, and hold the breath in for 4 counts. Release the ring finger and exhale through your left nostril, for 4 counts (Image #2).

Now inhale through the left nostril, 4 counts, hold your breath with both closed 4 counts, and exhale through the right nostril 4 counts.

When you have a pattern going, continue for *at least a full minute.*

It helps to rest for 30 seconds or more afterward, to enjoy the calm feeling and avoid dizziness as you return to activity.

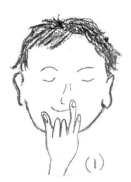
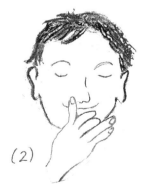

Note: *Illustration looks reversed because the person is facing you. Use your right hand, and start with ring finger over left nostril.*

Challengers !
Great for practicing focus and concentration.

Trace the Wheel
Can be done seated or standing.

Benefits: Improves alertness and concentration. Makes you laugh or smile, I hope. Synchronizes left and right hemispheres.

Actions: While seated, or standing with one foot a half-step in front and knees bent for stability:

(1) Reach your Right hand out in front of you, as if to shake someone's hand. Now imagine "tracing a wheel": your fingers point UP as they come in toward your chest, then DOWN as your hand moves outward, along the "wheel edge". Repeat the circling motion 3 more times. Easy.

(2) Now draw the wheel with your *Left hand only*... but the fingers go the *opposite way*. Left fingers point UP as they move <u>away</u> from you, and DOWN as they draw in toward you, to complete the circle. Practice circling the Left hand 3 or more times.

(3) *Your CHALLENGE:* Draw the wheel with both hands at once. Your fingers move in opposite directions: Right fingers point UP as they come IN towards your chest; and Left fingers point UP as they move OUT.

  With practice, it gets easier.

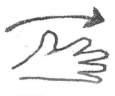

LEFT

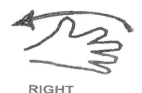

RIGHT

Climbing Spider – As in the "Itsy Bitsy Spider" song
(If you know the song, you could sing it as you go!)

Benefits: Aids concentration. Makes you laugh or smile (I hope). Synchronizes left and right hemispheres.

Actions:

(a) Touch your right index finger to your left thumb. (b) Keep them touching, and bring your right thumb to touch your left index finger. Now release contact (a) and "pivot" the hands around so the right index and left thumb meet again.

To create a "climbing" effect, keep pivoting at your contact points as shown. *Now it gets interesting:*

Do the same contacts with middle fingers to thumbs, several times… then ring finger to thumb, then pinky, and then back up the line to index finger again.

Whew! Spend at least a minute on this one.

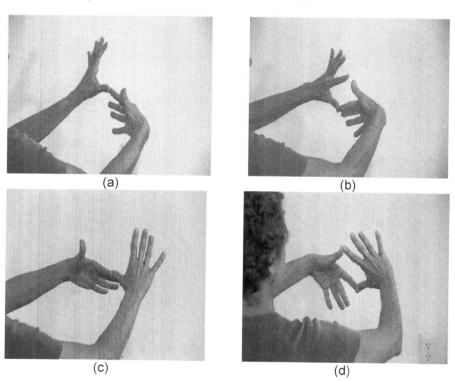

(a)　　　　　　　　　　(b)

(c)　　　　　　　　　　(d)

Eagle Pose - *A Balancing Act!*
Gentle version is shown in Photo 3.

Benefits: Calms and focuses your mind. Crossing your midline works your brain hemispheres in unison.

Actions: Begin by standing with feet about hip-width apart. Bend your knees as if preparing to sit. Lift right knee and cross right leg over the left. If possible, hook right foot behind left calf (Photo 2) OR let right foot hang by the side of left calf.

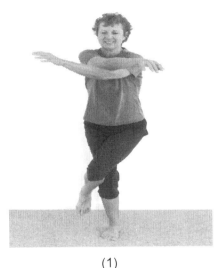

Tuck your right arm under your left arm and "wrap it around" if you can, bringing palms close together. Hold the posture for 5 breaths, and then do the same on the other side.

Adaptations (#3): Hug yourself and rest your toes down outside of your standing foot. You could also try the pose with your back or hip resting against a wall.

(1)

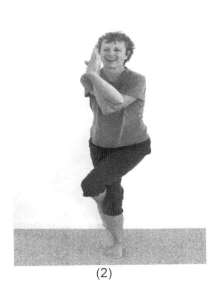

(2)

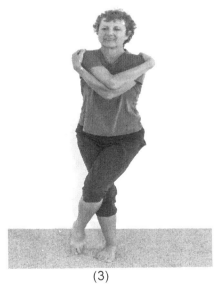

(3)

8's and 0's

Benefits: Improves focus and concentration. Makes you laugh or smile (I hope). Synchronizes left and right hemispheres.

Actions: As in "8's in the Sky" exercise, you're standing with feet shoulder-width apart. Raise your right arm to chest height. Draw a sideways figure 8 in the air with your right hand. Do this a few times, and then...

Your challenge: Draw a circle in the air with your left hand, while you draw the 8 with your right hand. Draw at least 4, and then change sides: do a circle with your right hand, and 8 with your left. Interesting?

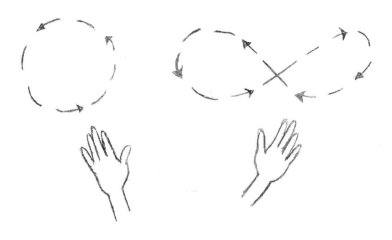

8's and 0's with Feet!

It's tough, but fun ... *Ready?*

Keep your abdominal muscles tight to avoid straining your back. While lying on your back or seated, lift both feet up to a comfortable height. Bend your knees, if you like.

Draw sideways 8's with your right foot while drawing 0's with your left. Switch sides and repeat. This works your abs, legs, and brain. *Enjoy.*

Thumb and Pinky

Benefits: Full brain activation; makes you concentrate and smile!
Actions: Hold your two fists up at about chest-height. Raise just your right thumb and left pinky finger. Then go back to fists. Raise just left thumb and right pinky, and then alternate, several times.
  Too easy? Try speeding up.

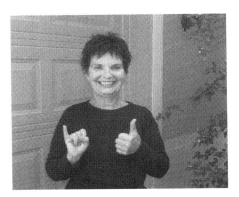 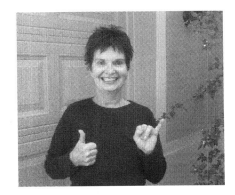

Expressing with "the other hand"

Benefits: Builds new circuits in the hemisphere that's normally less active when you write. Gets your creativity flowing... you might find new ideas popping up.
Actions: With your non-dominant hand, write or draw on any surface, or with a computer drawing program. Create any images you like. With regular practice, you can increase the coordination in this hand.

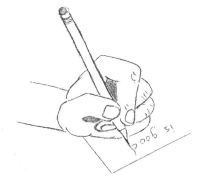

6

Summary of Exercises

Activators
These energizing, coordinated movements build and strengthen neural pathways, as the receptive and expressive areas of your brain work in unison.

Conscious Walking

Benefit: Provides awareness of your contra-lateral limb movements. Works the brain hemispheres in unison, just as normal walking does.

Actions: Take a walk – indoors or out – for at least 3 minutes, and note how your opposite-side arm naturally comes forward with each foot. This contra-lateral movement helps us balance as we walk.

Follow each breath flowing in and out, for a good mind-body connection. You may like to count your inhales and exhales.

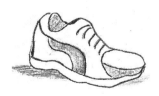

Depending on how fast you walk, for example, take 4 to 6 steps as you inhale, and 4 to 6 steps with each exhale.

Try swinging your arms more than usual. That's all you do in this "3-minute set".

> *"The sovereign invigorator of the body is exercise.*
> *And of all the exercises, walking is best."*
> -Thomas Jefferson

Same – Same

As mentioned earlier, you **only** need this homolateral movement if your energy is very low, and the crossovers feel like a struggle. Or try the "Bear Walk", in Chapter 4.

If we feel sluggish—our energy may be "stuck" - moving weakly up and down each side of the body, and not crossing center.

Do you ever feel "mentally foggy", first thing in the morning, or after sitting at the computer for hours? It may also occur after an illness or a long period of inactivity.[1,2]

Benefit: Moves your energy along homo-lateral lines, on either side of the body. (Gets it moving, so it will be easier to do the crossover moves!)

Actions: Standing with feet about hip-width apart, inhale and lift your left arm and left knee at the same time. As you exhale, lower the left arm and leg, and lift your right arm and leg. Go back and forth, slowly, for at least 8 lifts on each side. NOW you're ready for the Activator Exercises.

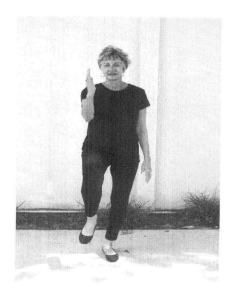 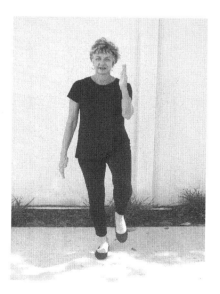

The brain is built to change in response to experience.
It's transformable. – Dr. Richard Davidson

Swingin' *(Easier than Crossovers on next page)*

Benefits: Both arms cross your midline at once, for whole brain activation. The twisting burns calories and trims your waistline.

Actions: With knees bent and feet about shoulder-width apart, enjoy swinging your arms. Let your hips sway, and weight shift side to side. As the arms cross your midline, touch left hip with right hand, and if possible, bring your left hand around behind you to touch the right hip. Keep swinging arms back and forth across midline, and tapping hips.

Breathe! Keep your shoulders relaxed, and go at least 30 seconds.

Adaptation: The arm movements can be done while seated.

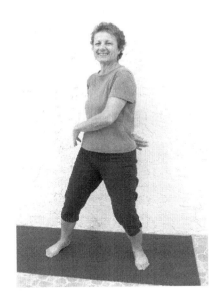 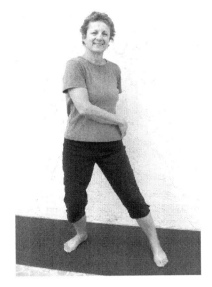

Believe you can and you're halfway there.
-Theodore Roosevelt

Crossover

(or try a Crossover Challenge, on next page)

Benefit: Crossing midline in a rhythmic pattern activates your two brain hemispheres in unison. You "switch your brain on" with these moves.

Actions: Stand with your feet about hip-width apart. Reach your left hand across to touch the right knee as you raise it, and then do the same with the right hand on the left knee. As if slowly "marching in place", continue for 30 seconds or more.

Adaptation: Can be done while seated.

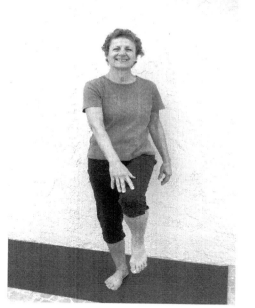 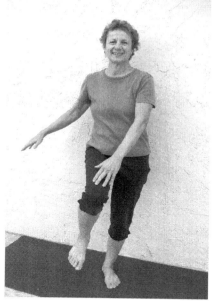

You can't push the river, but you can steer your boat.

Crossover Challenges

These challenge your balance and give you more of a twist. *Try one or more,* without forcing any stretches.

Benefits: Full brain activation by crossing your midline.

Actions:

Go at least 30 seconds, side to side, coordinating your breath with the movements:

(2) Cross over and touch right elbow to left knee, and then left elbow to right knee.

(2) Lift your foot and cross over to touch it. 3) Kick a foot up behind you. Reach behind with opposite side hand to touch it.

Adaptations: #1 and 2 can be done while seated. #3 could be done with a counter top or other sturdy support in front of you. Place one hand on the support.

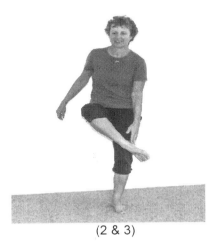

(2 & 3)

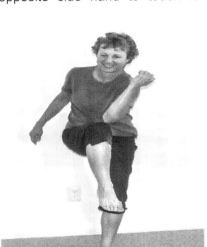

(1)

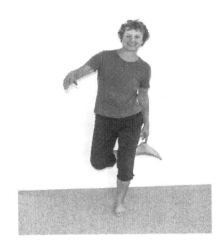

Beach Ball Twist

Benefits: Crossing midline stimulates nerve messages between brain hemispheres, so your receptive and expressive sides work together. Challenges your balance and tones the abdominals.

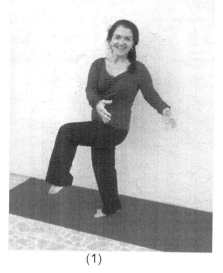
(1)

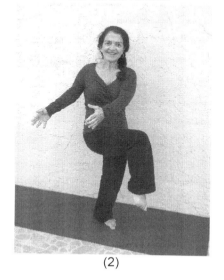
(2)

Actions: Imagine holding a beach ball at your right hip. Lift your right knee across your midline and point it to the left front corner. Optional: touch your right hip with left hand as you go. Come back to center, and repeat on the other side. Go back and forth, tossing 8 times to each side.

BREATHE with the movements, exhaling on the toss. Enjoy.

Adaptations: You could hold a sturdy support with one hand, while "tossing back" with the other.

If lifting your knee is a problem, just cross one straight leg in front of the other and tap the toe down in front.

A mind unshaken by worldly states…
This is the Blessing Supreme.
- Buddha

Laugh It Up!

"There's a real science to this, and it's as real as taking a drug."
Lee Berk, M.D., Professor of Medicine, Loma Linda Univ.[3]

Having fun with friends and family often gets us laughing, but for an extra shot of joy, here are three suggested activities.

Read more about the power of laughter in Chapter Nine.

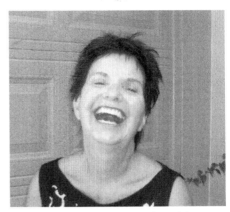

Mary Lou loves to laugh!

Benefits: Laughing releases endorphins, the neurotransmitters that boost a positive state of mind and reduce stress.

Actions: Yes, these *are silly* exercises. That's the idea! Hopefully they will result in genuine laughter, to brighten your day.

Do them with a BIG smile, in front of a mirror, or with friends.

(1) Take a deep breath, and as you exhale, say "Huh!" Bring the sound out from deep in your belly. Repeat several times, then change "huh" to "ha!" Go through all the vowel sounds: Hee, hee! Hih (like the "i" in "pin") Hih, Hih! Heh, Heh, Hoo, Hoo!

(2) While clapping hands, say "Ho, ho. Ha, ha, ha!" Clap in time with the beat you create. You could use background music and follow the beat. Try various vowel sounds: "Hee, hee, hee! Ha, ha, hah!" Point at yourself in the mirror, or at your friends. Go at least 30 seconds.

Next, hold a grin for **at least** 10 seconds, and then raise arms in a big "V" and say, "Very good, very good—Yay! Laugh and clap another 30 seconds. Now you're feeling great!

(3) Use hats, a clown nose, or any costumes that get the giggles going. Surprise someone by showing up in costume. Make eye contact, take a deep breath, and exhale with "Aah, ha, ha, ha!" Go at least a full minute.

How long does it take for *your* fake laughter to become real?

Smile!

As recommended by "the Laugh Doctor", Cliff Kuhn, M.D.

Benefits: Smiling boosts your mood and energy as it activates endorphins, "the feel-good chemicals" in your brain. Dr. Kuhn has prescribed it for hundreds of depressed patients, and he says those willing to practice it "always report mood elevation and a reduction in symptoms—almost instantly!" [4]

Your brain doesn't know the difference between a fake smile and genuine smile. I used "smiling on purpose" while driving to class on a few cold, dark Alaskan mornings. My students were lucky...I showed up in a great mood!

Actions: Curl up the edges of your mouth, show your teeth, and hold that smile...for at least 20 to 30 seconds.

This can be done any time, of course, for as long as you like.

Read more about brain benefits of smiling and laughing in Chapter 9.

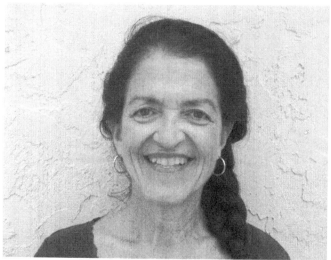

Thanks for the smiles, Angela!

A happy, positive expression will serve you well in life.
- Jennifer Smith

V for Vitality

Benefits: Opens the lungs for enhanced breathing. Crossing your arms stimulates nerve messaging for full-brain activation.

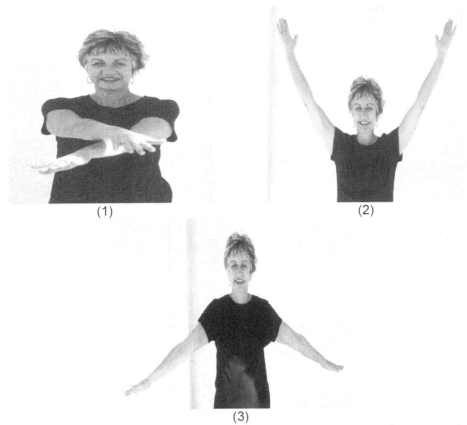

(1) (2) (3)

Actions: Stand with feet shoulder-width apart. Raise both arms out in front of you. Cross forearms, and then lift and separate them, like a "V". Breathe in as you lift and open the arms. Breathe out as you bring them down by your sides.

Repeat, alternating the arm on top, for a total of 8 circles.

Adaptation: May be done in a chair. If your shoulders feel strained, try lifting your arms just halfway up.

"The Eyes Have It"

The next four exercises involve your eyes in keeping your brain happy.

Drawing 8's with eyes

Benefits: "Switches the brain on" for energy and mental clarity, as it stimulates messaging between hemispheres. Refreshes tired eyes.

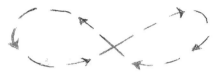

Actions: While seated or lying down, *keep your eyes closed* and draw sideways figure 8's (the infinity symbol) with your eyes. Notice the "X" in the center of the 8 ... this increases nerve messaging between hemispheres.

Draw them 4 or 5 times one way, and then reverse direction. Smile!

Refresh your eyes

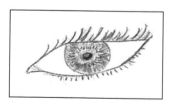

Benefits: Relieves stress and enhances circulation in your eyes.
Actions: While sitting or lying down, rub your palms together briskly to create some heat. Close your eyes and gently cover them with your palms. Rest your fingers on your forehead and take 3 deep, relaxing breaths.

Third Eye (Brow Point) Gazing

This is a focusing technique that may help in meditation. Take care not to strain your eyes.

It's been said that gazing at the brow point balances the pineal gland in the brain. Located at the top of the spinal cord where the head and neck are joined, this gland affects the body's hormones. Ancient yogic texts of India refer to the pineal gland as "the eye of intuition" or "third eye". This gland has striking similarities to our eyes, with pigmented, retinal cells surrounding a chamber of globular lens-like mass.[5]

Benefit: Synchronizes the two brain hemispheres. Calms and connects mind and body.

Actions: Sit comfortably and *close your eyes* or leave them slightly open. Look up toward the space between your eyebrows, then a little higher. Beginners could place one or two fingers here on your forehead so you feel "where to look." Keep your gaze in this direction. If your eyes feel strained, bring them back to normal, and perhaps try again later with eyes a little higher or lower.

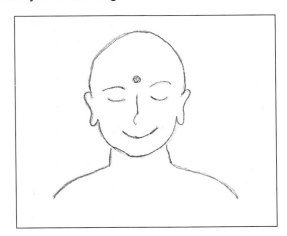

Hold the gaze for at least 30 seconds. Breathe deeply for a few breaths, then return to normal mindful breathing. When your mind wanders, bring it back to the breath. You might decide to make this a regular practice, for longer periods of time.

Adaptation: May be done lying on your back.

Columns

Benefit: "Switches the brain on" for energy and mental clarity, as nerve messages travel between the two hemispheres. Research conducted at Manchester Metropolitan University in England has shown that repeated horizontal eye movements can have a positive effect on memory.[6]

Actions: With eyes closed, picture two vertical columns. The left one has letters going down it: A,B,C,D, and E. The right column has numbers going down, from 1 through 5. Visualize enough space between your columns so your eyes must move side to side in this exercise.

Smile, keep your eyes closed, and:
Look back and forth from left to right, counting:
A-1, B-2, etc... to E-5.
Now reverse direction, from right to left, picturing:
1-A, 2-B ... to 5-E.
Rest your eyes for a few breaths. Repeat at least once more.

A ----------------------------------- 1

B ----------------------------------- 2

C ----------------------------------- 3

D ----------------------------------- 4

E ----------------------------------- 5

Life can only be understood backwards,
But it must be lived forwards.
Soren Kierkegaard

Create A Happy Scene

Benefits: Releases endorphins to reduce stress and enhance mood; regular practice helps you achieve positive goals.

Actions: Relax in a comfortable place, close your eyes and imagine a movie screen six inches out from your face, and an inch or more above your eye level. Although most people make pictures in the forehead between the eyebrows, psychologist and author Rita Milios says placing your mind's movie screen comfortably out in space "allows you to relax and have more spontaneous creative images." [7]

Create a scene on your "movie screen." Depending on your goal in this exercise, you might imagine a serene natural setting, or see yourself in a successful business meeting, or enjoying time with friends / family, etc.

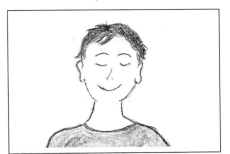

Use all your senses in the imagery: what are you seeing, hearing, tasting, touching and smelling? How do you feel? What are you and others saying? Get into the scene, as if you are "in the movie."

Smile and continue your "movie of the mind" for a few minutes.

Exhale!

Breathe only as deeply as is comfortable, to avoid dizziness.

Benefits: A deep, "complete" exhale removes old, stale air trapped in your lungs. Energizes you, with a good dose of fresh, clean air.

Action: *Lying on your back*, inhale deeply. Now purse your lips like you're whistling and slowly blow all the air out, sinking your belly down toward your spine. Even when you think all the air is gone, try to push out a little more. Then feel the clean, refreshing air filling your lungs on the next inhale.

Practice the full exhale at least twice. Then relax with normal breathing a while, before sitting or standing up.

If you get light-headed, stop and rest, lying down and breathing normally for a few minutes. You may want to try it another time.

8's in the Sky

Benefits: Activates left and right hemispheres in unison; limbers the shoulders and enhances your breathing.

Actions: Stand with your knees slightly bent and your feet shoulder-width apart, for a solid stance. Raise your right arm straight out in front of you, at chest height. Draw a big sideways figure 8 in the air with your right hand.

Tips:

Drawing upward through the center of your "8", as Dr. Hannaford suggests, follows energy flowing up the midline of your body.

Focusing on the "X" at center of the "8" engages neural pathways across the corpus callosum, and synchronizes brain hemispheres.[8]

Make the 8 wider than your shoulders and higher than your head, to really work your arms and get hemispheres engaged.

As you move, let your weight shift a little, from side to side.

Draw it 5 times with your right hand, then 5 times with your left.

Now draw it 5 times with both hands, one resting on the other.

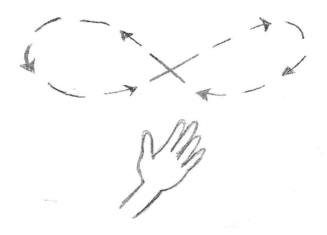

Normal day, let me be aware of the treasure that you are.
Mary Jean Irion

Climbing Spider – *Like the "Itsy Bitsy Spider" song.*
(If you know the song, you could sing it as you go!)

Benefits: Improves alertness and concentration. Makes you laugh or smile, I hope. Synchronizes left and right hemispheres.

Actions:
   (a) Touch your right index finger to your left thumb. (b) Keep them touching, and bring your right thumb to touch your left index finger. Now release contact (a) and "pivot" the hands around so the right index and left thumb meet again.
   To create a "climbing" effect, keep pivoting at your contact points.

Now it gets interesting:
Do the same contacts with middle fingers to thumbs, several times… then ring finger to thumb, then pinky, and then back up the line to index finger again.
   Whew! Spend at least a minute on this one.

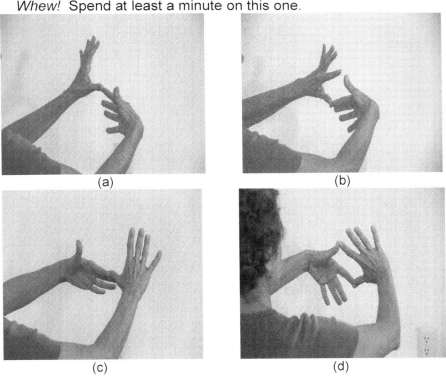

(a)　　　　　　　　　　　　(b)

(c)　　　　　　　　　　　　(d)

Using Your "Other Hand"

Benefit: Using your non-dominant hand accesses right brain functions, *regardless* of which hand we favor. This is explained by Lucia Cappachione in *The Power of Your Other Hand.*[9]

Musicians who use both hands have about a nine percent increase in the size of their corpus callosum, which connects the two hemispheres, according to research noted by Dr. Carl Hale, neuropsychologist. This increased exchange can benefit information processing, he says.[10]

Like a TV set, your brain receives information from elsewhere, adds Cappachione. The left brain, being logical and methodical, gets standard local channels, while the right brain is like "subscribing to cable or satellite service." It tunes in to more feelings, creativity and inner wisdom.[11]

Actions: Try some everyday activities with your non-dominant hand. Use the toothbrush, computer mouse, TV remote, doorknobs, eating utensils, etc., with your "other hand."

(1) Draw with Both Hands

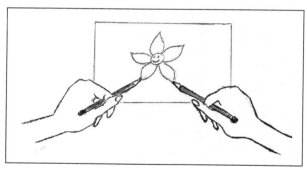

Actions: On a chalkboard, dry erase board, or paper, draw a simple image with both hands at once: a house, tree, flower, face, etc.

Move both hands at once. Try using a different colored pen or chalk in each hand. ***Experiment and play.*** ☺ You could keep the hands parallel and draw a symmetrical flower, or move the markers in different directions simultaneously. Smile! Share this one with the kids.

(2) Draw with "the other hand"

Benefits: Builds neural circuits in the hemisphere that you normally don't use often in drawing or writing. Boosts your creativity.
Actions: With your non-dominant hand, draw on any surface, or with a computer drawing program. Create any images you like. With regular practice, you can increase the coordination of movements in this hand.

Notice how you feel after this drawing.

(3) Write with "the other hand"

Benefits: A new way of looking at things may arise, as you get your logical side out of the way.

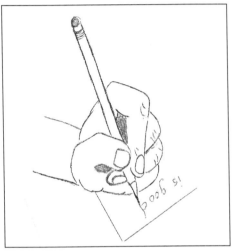

Full-brain activation occurs as messages travel between your brain hemispheres.

Don't worry about how this handwriting looks! Go slowly, and allow your creative side to flourish.

Is there a problem clouding your mind? Try writing about it with your "other hand" and see if a creative solution pops up.

Actions: Spend a few minutes writing in a notebook or on paper, with your non-dominant hand. Try "long-hand" cursive writing, as well as printing. At first you could write larger than your usual size, if this makes it more legible. *Enjoy.*

I am much more interested in being creative than in being busy.
Creating feels good.
- Bernie Siegel

8's and 0's

Benefits: Increases your focus and concentration. Makes you laugh or smile, I hope. Synchronizes left and right hemispheres.

Actions: As in 8's in the Sky, you're standing with feet shoulder-width apart. Raise your right arm to chest height. Draw a sideways figure 8 in the air with your right hand. Do this a few times, and then *your challenge is to:*

Draw a circle in the air with your left hand, while you draw the 8 with your right hand. Draw at least 4, and then change sides: do a circle with your right hand, and sideways 8 with your left. Interesting? Repeat the sequence at least once more.

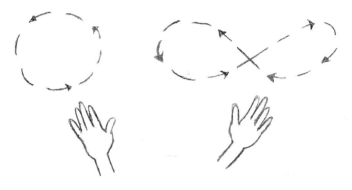

8's and 0's with Feet!

It's tough, but fun ... *Ready?*

Keep your abdominal muscles tight to avoid straining your back. While lying on your back, lift both feet in the air to a comfortable height. Draw sideways 8's with your right foot while drawing 0's with your left. Switch sides and repeat. Works your <u>abs</u>, legs, and brain. *Enjoy.*

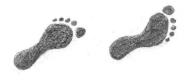

Seated Twist

Benefits: Relieves spinal tension and refreshes organs / glands. Crossing midline helps activate neural pathways, as your brain hemispheres work in unison.

Actions: Sitting up tall, place your left hand on your right knee.

Turn and look left, breathe normally and with each exhale, relax into the twist. Hold for 3 breaths.

Change sides and repeat, then do one more twist on each side.

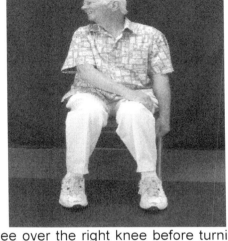

Adaptation: For more twisting (and brain benefit) cross left knee over the right knee before turning to your left, and cross right knee over left knee, before turning right.

Go Fly a Kite!

This old English idiom means "go away and leave me alone." I'm using it here with a different twist, meaning "get away from your daily tasks, put the freight train of your thoughts in neutral, and do something for the sheer pleasure of it!"

Brains thrive with activities that are interesting, challenging, and new. Nourish yours by doing something *fun*.

Get outdoors and enjoy nature (or fly a kite), listen to music, take a walk in a new place, try a new puzzle or game with the kids …

There is no time limit for this exercise. *Whether it's one minute or a whole day, you will benefit.*

Seated Side Stretch

Benefits: Crossing midline with both arms at once; this stretch relieves tension in hips and back, opens the lungs and increases your energy with improved circulation.

Actions:
Sitting up tall, with right hand on your left thigh. Keep the hip down on your left side, and raise your left arm, reaching over your head toward the right wall. Hold for a few breaths, and then change sides. Repeat once more on each side.

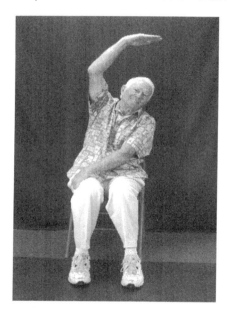 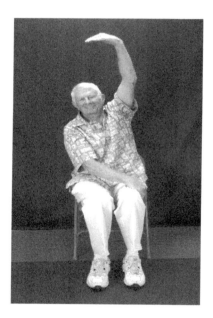

How high you can go is mostly a matter of where you set your sights.
- U.S. Anderson

Thumb and Pinky

Benefits: Full brain activation; makes you concentrate and smile!
Actions: Hold your two fists up at about chest-height. Raise just your right thumb and left pinky finger. Then go back to fists. Raise just left thumb and right pinky, and then alternate, several times.
   Too easy? Try speeding up.

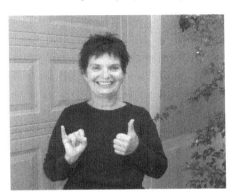 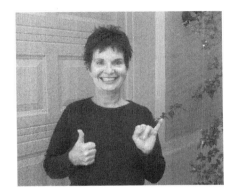

Hand Clasp

Benefits: Crossing your fingers in a new pattern is like writing with your non-dominant hand: it builds and enhances neural pathways.[12]
Actions: Clasp your hands together naturally and rest them on a

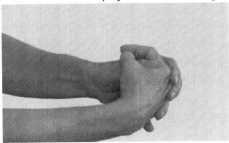

table or desk. Notice how one thumb is above the other, one forefinger on top of the other, and so on. Now separate your hands and re-clasp, with the other thumb and fingers on top.

Hold this clasp; let each exhale wash tension away from your body/mind. Squeeze the fingers a little tighter together for a few seconds, to be aware of this unique connection. Do a gentle "squeeze and release" every 10 to 15 seconds, as you hold the clasp about 1 minute.

Trace the Wheel

Can be done seated or standing; it gets easier with practice.

Benefits: Aids focus and concentration. Makes you laugh or smile (I hope). Synchronizes left and right brain hemispheres.

Actions:
(1) Reach your Right hand out in front of you, as if to shake someone's hand. Now imagine "tracing a wheel": your fingers point UP as they come in toward your chest, then DOWN as your hand moves outward, along the "wheel edge". Repeat the circling motion 3 more times. Easy.
(2) Now draw the wheel with your *Left hand only*... but the fingers go the *opposite way*. Left fingers point UP as they move <u>away</u> from you, and DOWN as they draw in toward you, to complete the circle. Circle the Left hand 3 or more times.
(3) *Your CHALLENGE:* Draw the wheel with both hands at once. Your fingers move in opposite directions: Right fingers point UP as they come IN, and Left fingers point UP as they move OUT. *Enjoy!*

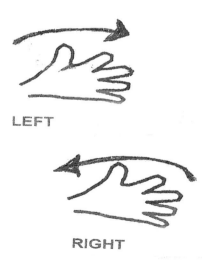

LEFT

RIGHT

The most common form of despair is not being who you are.
Soren Kierkegaard

Juggling!

Currently, I can barely juggle two tennis balls. I hope to master three, after I finish this book project!

Benefits: Eye-hand coordination. Crossing of midline with eyes creates whole brain activation. Makes you laugh, I hope.

Actions: If you're experienced at juggling, you might enjoy including it in your brain-building workouts.

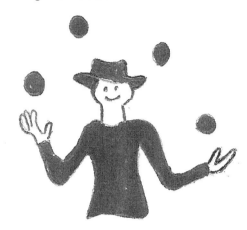

If you're new to juggling: start with just one tennis ball (or other small ball, or a bean bag). While standing or seated, toss the ball back and forth between hands, keeping it around eye level.

When you are comfortable with this, try two balls. With one in each hand, toss a ball from your less dominant hand to your dominant hand. (The dominant hand feels stronger and more adept at tossing and catching.)

Just before you catch the ball in your dominant hand, throw the other ball you are holding, to the less dominant hand.

Yes, you will drop balls, many times. *Keep working at it!*

Ready to try three balls? Visit the website noted below, where you can get free lessons. Some people learn to juggle in one day. Others might need several weeks. As explained on the site, practice and persistence are keys to success.

   Enjoy!

http://www.learnhowtojuggle.info

Sa Ta Na Ma

Based in Kundalini Yoga, this exercise involves repeating sounds and finger poses (mudras). The Sanskrit syllables Sa, Ta, Na, Ma translate as birth, life, death, and rebirth.

Benefits: Increases circulation in the brain, promotes focus, clarity, and mind-body-spirit connection, according to Philameana lila Desy, author of *The Everything Guide to Reiki.*[13]

Actions: Sitting upright, recite "Sa Ta Na Ma" while pressing the thumb with alternating fingertips. You can use one hand at a time, or both hands at the same time. Keep repeating in a stable rhythm, pressing the thumb with:

SA—index finger.
TA—middle finger.
NA—ring finger.
MA—small finger.

Continue at least one minute, for the best effect.

Some Kundalini Yoga teachers will continue for 11 or 31 minutes, following their tradition.

Find more information at these websites:

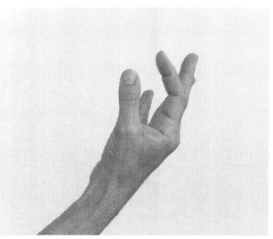

http://healing.about.com/b/2012/04/03/sa-ta-na-ma-meditation.html
http://www.kundaliniyoga.org/kyt15.html

The point of power is always in the present moment.
- Louise Hay

Refreshers

These exercises and postures help to focus and calm your body/mind. They replenish your energy and vitality.

"Dissolving" Pose

Relaxation is the final posture in most yoga classes. The Sanskrit word for it is "Savasana". *Sava* means dissolve, and *Asana* means posture.

Benefits: Deep relaxation reduces the stress hormones cortisol and noradrenaline, decreases the rate of aging, and increases an attitude of acceptance, says Dr. Herbert Benson, Harvard University professor and author of *The Relaxation Response.*[14]

Actions: Lying on your back, deeply exhale at least once: draw your belly button down toward your spine as you push all your air out through pursed lips. Feel the clean, refreshing air filling your lungs on the inhale. Then take a few slow, deep breaths, if you wish.

Now breathe normally, feeling how your abdomen lifts and lowers, the rib cage expands, the air moves in your nostrils. Observe your sensations with every breath. You could focus on just one, i.e., your nostrils, or notice all sensations, including the sound of your breath.

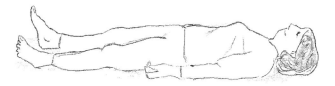

Feel your muscles "letting go" on each exhale, as tension dissolves away. Release any concerns. Focus on the calm stillness; feel your weight resting on the floor or bed. Relax completely for at least one full minute.

Come out of the resting pose slowly and mindfully.

Feelings come and go, like clouds in a windy sky. Conscious breathing is my anchor. –Thich Nhat Hahn

Balancing Circle

Adapted from a Tai Chi exercise called Prayer Wheel, or Tracing the Drum. Your fingers draw a circle, as in "Trace the Wheel".

Hint: Focusing your gaze on one small spot in front of you may make it easier to balance on one leg.

Benefits: Activates your vestibular system and gives you practice in balancing. Strengthens and tones your legs.

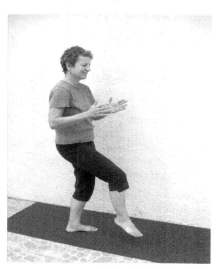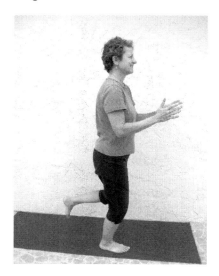

Actions: Stand with feet hip width apart. Place your right foot forward, about a step and a half. Keep your back tall, and shoulders relaxed.

With both feet flat, shift your weight forward and back from right to left foot, while bending and straightening your knees.

Hands are about six inches apart; palms face each other. Draw a circle with your fingertips, as if tracing the edges of a wheel or drum. Sink weight back into your left foot as your fingertips come up and in toward you; then shift weight forward onto your right foot as fingertips go down and outward.

If you feel stable, start a rocking motion. Lift one foot at a time, about 10 inches off the ground, but even a few inches will be effective.

Do 8 wheels with right foot forward, then 8 more with left foot forward. If this exercise is helpful, do another round of 8 on each side.

Adaptation: You can hold a sturdy support with one hand, and draw the wheel with your other hand.

Tree Pose

This posture can be basic (as shown) or highly challenging, depending on where you place your raised foot and arms. Enjoy creating your tree.

Benefits: Activates your vestibular system as you balance on one leg and both sides of the brain work in unison. Helps calm and focus the mind, and strengthen your legs.

Actions: Imagine your right foot has deep roots sinking into the ground. Raise your left leg, bending the knee and placing the sole of the foot on the right leg: by the ankle, calf, or against the thigh.

Find a comfortable arm/hand position. You could try raising arms above your head.

Hold the posture for 4 breaths, and then repeat on the other side.

Adaptation: Rest your standing hip (or a hand) on a sturdy support.

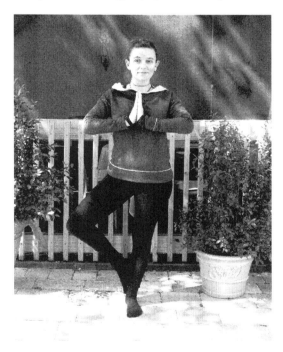

Life is a balancing act.

"Hands Float Like Clouds" – A Tai Chi exercise

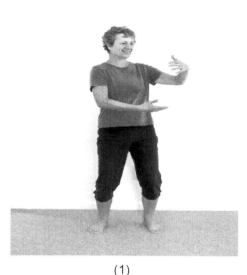

Benefits: Helps to calm and focus the mind, as breathing goes with the moves. Nerve messages travel between brain hemispheres as arms cross your body's midline.

Keep in Mind: Relaxing arms, hands and wrists, for a soft, "fluid" feeling.

Your arms remain still, going with your torso as you turn at the waist.

What may help: Have someone read the instructions aloud, the first few times you do this one. It seems complex at first, and yet it's simple and graceful.

(1)

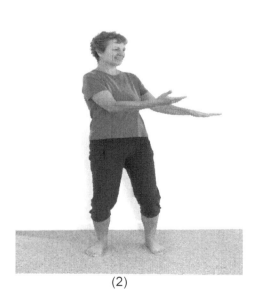

(2)

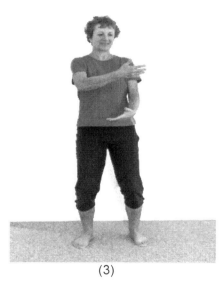

(3)

Hands Float Like Clouds, *continued*

Actions: Stand with your feet about shoulder-width apart, toes turned slightly outward. Bend your knees, for a solid stance.

Imagine holding a basketball in front of your chest. Your left hand is under it and right hand is behind it, facing you.

Left palm is facing up, at chest level. Right hand is about 6 inches above it, with palm facing toward your chin (photo 1).

Keeping your arms still, turn slowly toward your right until you're facing the right front corner (45-degree turn). Gradually switch hands (photo 2).

Now your right hand is under the ball, and left is up behind the ball (at chin level). (photo 3). Turn slowly to the left, keeping arms still, until you're facing your left front corner. (photo 4) Change hands and begin turning to your right again (photo 5).

Continue back and forth, *breathing in as you turn one way, and out as you turn the other way.*

Feel your hands "floating like clouds". Do this exercise for *at least* 2 minutes. It takes about a minute to settle the mind into the body, and then you'll enjoy the flow.

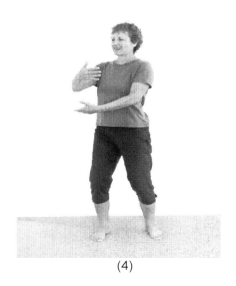

(4)

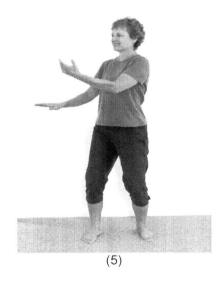

(5)

Cow & Cat

Benefits: Enhances energy, metabolism and a positive mood, as tucking chin toward chest stimulates your thyroid gland. More blood reaches the brain through this exercise. It works all the spinal muscles, increases circulation and relieves tension in your back and neck.

Actions: Start in tabletop position: hands just below shoulders, and knees below your hips. Round your spine upward for Cat Pose (like a frightened cat). Tuck your chin gently toward your chest. (Photo 1) Hold for two breaths, then slowly sink your spine downward for cow pose. (Photo 2) You may want to lift your chin and sit bones for more curve in the spine. Do not force the stretch. Hold for two breaths, then go back and forth at your own pace, inhaling in cow pose and exhaling in cat pose.

Adaptation: May be done seated in a chair, or cross-legged on the floor. Relax your shoulders; curve the spine forward for "cow" and back for "cat". Lifting and lowering your chin is optional.

Share it with the kids! Smile and enjoy.

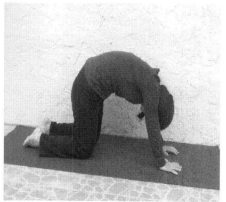 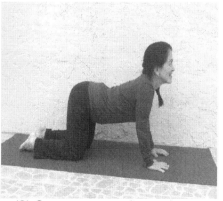

| (2) Cat Pose – arched spine with chin tucked. | (2) Cow pose – sunken spine |

Let the child in you come out and play!

Eagle Pose   *Think: Pretzel !*
  Gentle version is shown in Photo 3.

Benefits: Stretches shoulders and opens upper back; calms and focuses your mind. Crossing midline activates both hemispheres.

Actions: Begin by standing with feet about hip-width apart. Bend your knees as if preparing to sit. Lift right knee and cross right leg

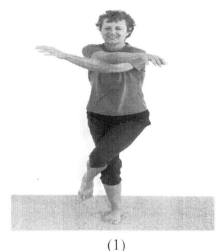

over the left. If possible, hook right foot behind left calf (Photo 2) OR let right foot hang by the side of left calf.

Tuck your right arm under your left arm and "wrap it around" if you can, bringing palms close together. Hold the posture for 5 breaths, and then do the same on the other side.

***Adaptations** (# 3):* Hug yourself and rest your toes down outside of your standing foot. You could also try the pose with your back or hip resting against a wall.

(1)

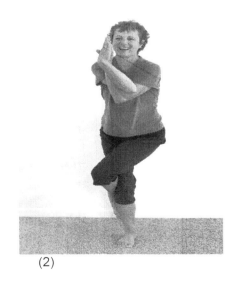

(2)

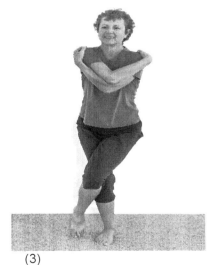

(3)

Downward Dog Pose

Using a yoga mat will prevent your hands and feet from slipping.

In this classic yoga pose, your head is below your heart, so more blood reaches the brain.

Benefits: Calms the nervous system. Relieves tension in neck, shoulders and spinal column. Stretches hamstrings, calves, and arms for energy, circulation, and muscle tone.

Stretching your calf muscles aids the ability to follow through and complete projects, according to Brain Gym® [15]

Actions: On hands and knees with your hands slightly forward of your shoulders, turn your toes under and lift your hips up high; reach your heels toward the floor, but they don't have to touch it. Press your chest back toward your thighs, so you have a long, straight spine. Relax neck and shoulders, with your head between your upper arms. Stay in dog pose for several breaths. Rest and repeat.

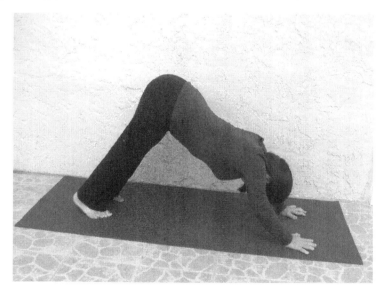

Downward Dog Pose. Relax shoulders and smile!

Deep Breathing

This is a three-part breath. You can take in seven times as much oxygen in this breath as you do in a shallow breath, says Swami Karunananda, senior instructor of Integral Yoga.[16]

Benefits: Energizes you with fresh oxygen reaching the brain and vital organs through your bloodstream. Expands your lower lungs as the diaphragm lowers on each inhale.

Actions: *Lie on your back* with knees bent and feet flat on the floor (or bed), hip-width apart. Picture your abdomen and chest as a balloon filling from the bottom up as you inhale.

First your abdomen expands, then the rib cage, and third is the upper chest. On your exhale, it follows the same order: first the abdomen sinks back down, then the rib cage and the chest. Finally, pull your abdomen in slightly to empty the lungs completely.

Beginners: try a 3-part breath slowly, two or three times, then pause for several normal breaths, and do a few more. If you feel dizzy, rest before standing up again.

Experienced breathers may take 5 or 6 breaths; rest and repeat.

Adaptations: May be done in a chair, but you'll feel more rising and falling, and have less possibility of dizziness while lying down.

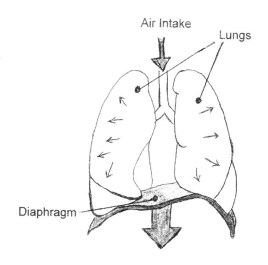

Air Intake

Lungs

Diaphragm

Mindful Breathing

Benefit: Brings calm and focus to a chattering mind
Actions: Sitting comfortably (or lying down) and smiling, feel the breath flowing in and out of your nostrils. Feel your ribcage expand on each inhale, and your whole body releasing with each exhale. Notice the pause—a moment of calm stillness—after each exhale, just before the next inhale. Relax and enjoy mindful breathing for about one minute.

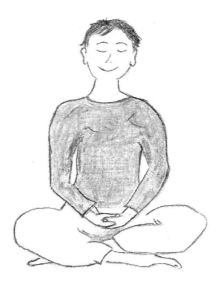

Options: (1) Keep a slight smile going in this exercise, to increase your brain benefits. (2) With eyes closed, look up toward your brow-point (known as the "3rd eye"), an area on your forehead that is midway between the eyebrows and a half-inch or so above. This technique helps me focus in meditation. It takes some practice before it feels comfortable.

> *"Being with the breath is the place where you feel at home."*
> - Thanissaro Bikkhu

Alternate Nostril Breath
This brain-balancing, calming technique is based in Yoga.

Everyone has a "nasal cycle" of air flowing predominantly through one nostril for about one to three hours, then switching to the other side, according to the National Institutes of Health.[17]

Benefits: Lowers the heart rate; reduces stress and anxiety.[18] Synchronizes the two brain hemispheres.[19]

Before starting: Read all of the Actions and the note below pictures.

Actions: Sitting with a tall spine, use the *right thumb and ring finger* to gently close off one nostril at a time. Curl your right index and middle finger down into your palm, so just the ring and pinky fingers are up.

Press your ring finger over your left nostril and inhale for 4 counts through your right nostril. Close your right nostril with your thumb, so both are now closed, and hold the breath in for 4 counts. Release the ring finger and exhale through your left nostril, for 4 counts.

Now inhale through the left nostril 4 counts, hold your breath with both closed 4 counts, and exhale through the right nostril 4 counts.

After you get the pattern established, continue for *at least a full minute.*

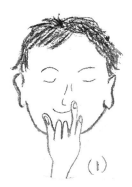 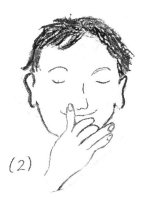

Note: *Illustration looks reversed because the person is facing you. Use your right hand, and start with ring finger over left nostril.*

Mindful Walking (a meditation)

This movement is slower and more deliberate than the Conscious Walking exercise. Mindful Walking helps us remember our connection with the Earth.

Benefits: Reduces stress; links mind and body in present moment awareness; with practice, enhances clarity and concentration.[20]
Actions: Find a place where you won't be disturbed for at least 5 minutes. Walk back and forth in a line, at least 15 feet long, or on a quiet path in nature.

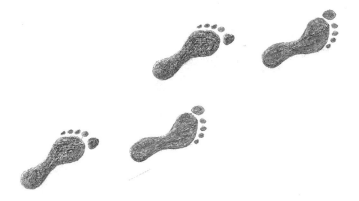

Walk VERY slowly, focusing on all your sensations. Follow each breath, and your foot lifting, moving and resting down with each step. Your mind will wander, but keep bringing it back to this experience.

You could repeat a mental phrase to keep the mind focused, such as "lifting, placing" or "left, right" or "I have arrived; I am home." It feels good to be at home in the now.

With one step, "I have arrived" and as the next foot settles in, "I am home." Coordinate your breathing with the steps in a comfortable rhythm. Enjoy mindful walking for a few minutes or more.

Present moment, joyful moment.
-Thich Nhat Hahn

Energy Link

I'm sitting on the floor in this photo…you could also sit in a chair or lie on your back.

Benefits: Has a calming effect, as it activates the vestibular system to increase focus and balance.

Actions: While seated or lying down, cross your ankles and make a pyramid shape with your hands—the pads of fingers and thumbs are touching. Press them together gently. Rest the tip of your tongue on the roof of your mouth, relax and breathe deeply a few times. Now return to normal breathing, holding the posture for at least 30 seconds more.

Adaptations: For a more powerful "energy linking" pose, try the next one, called "Hook-Ups.®"

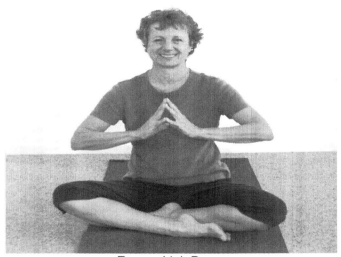
Energy Link Pose

Whoever is happy will make others happy too.
- Anne Frank

Hook-Ups®

Benefits: This Brain Gym® posture invites calm, while focusing and organizing scattered attention.[21] It brings attention to the motor cortex of your frontal hemispheres and away from the survival center in the back brain, thus decreasing adrenalin.[22]

Actions: Sitting with your back supported, or lying on your back:

Cross your ankles. It doesn't matter which is on top.

Extend your arms in front of you, and cross one wrist over the other.

Interlace your fingers and draw your clasped hands up toward your chest.

Hold like this for a minute or more, breathing slowly, with your eyes open or closed. As you inhale, touch the tip of your tongue to the roof of your mouth at the hard palate (just behind the teeth) and relax your tongue on exhalation.

Part Two *(NOT pictured)*: When ready, uncross your arms and legs and put your fingertips together in front of your chest, continuing to breathe deeply for another minute, and hold the tip of your tongue on the roof of your mouth when you inhale.

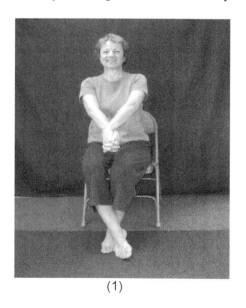

(1)

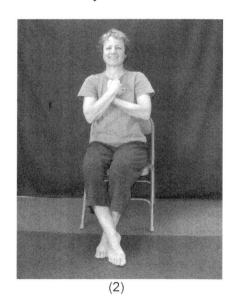

(2)

Pressure Points :

GB 20, Gates of Consciousness

Benefits: Regulates circulation to the brain and relaxes the nervous system. Pressing these points helps relieve a stiff neck, insomnia, headache and fatigue. It releases endorphins, the body's natural pain-killers, observes Michael Reed Gach, author of *Acupressure's Potent Points.*[23]

Location: In the hollows just under the base of the skull (occipital bone), on either side of your cervical spine.

Actions: Take a few deep breaths, as you press into these hollows, which are about three inches apart. Tilt your head back slowly and use your thumbs, fingers, or knuckles to gradually apply steady pressure. Hold for one to two minutes, relaxing and breathing with awareness.

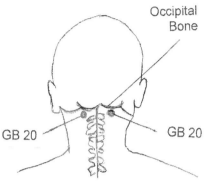

K-27, End points of the kidney meridians.

Benefits: Increases the flow of blood to your brain and gets your energy moving, so you feel more alert and positive.[24]

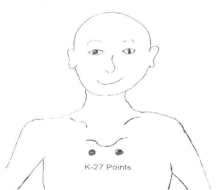

Location: Just under the collarbone. Place your fingertips on the U-shaped notch at the top of the breastbone, about where a man knots his tie. Then move them out and down about an inch, small depressions there.

Actions: Tap or hold steady pressure on the K-27 points with your two index fingers. Or just use one hand, touching the points with thumb and forefinger. Take a few deep breaths as you tap or hold the points
Rest for 30 seconds or more.

The Thinking Cap ®

This gets "head-turning" results in my classes! (Pun intended.)

Several brain benefits are gained in this exercise. Cecilia Koester, M.Ed., says 98% of those who try it report marked improvement in how far they can turn their heads.[25]

In Traditional Chinese Medicine, acupuncture points on the ears are noted for connecting large nerves to the brain.[26] The Thinking Cap helps relax tension in the neck and bring attention to the auditory system.[27]

One of my class members uses this before playing golf or backing up his car. He says he gets about 20% more head "turn-ability".

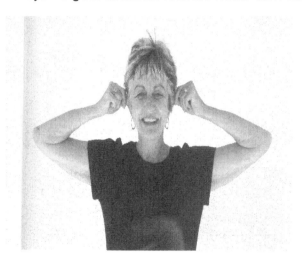

Actions: First, turn your head to the left and see how far you can look without straining your neck. Set a visual marker, like a doorknob. This is how far to the left you can look. Do the same on the right side, setting your visual marker.

Use your thumbs and index fingers to pull your ears gently back and unroll them. Begin at the top of the ear and massage down and around the curve, ending with the bottom lobe. Repeat 3 or more times.

Now, turn your head to the left and notice how far you can look. Is it past your marker? Then turn and check the right marker.

I hope you find it effective.

Standing Forward Bend

Benefits: Calms the brain; helps relieve stress, mild depression, headache and insomnia, according to Yoga Journal.[28]

Caution: If you feel too much pressure in your eyes or head, do not stay in the forward fold; slowly return to standing.

Actions: Standing up tall, bend forward from the hip joints (from the crease at the top of your legs. This keeps your spine straighter and torso longer than if you curl forward from the waist.) Let your arms dangle, or cross forearms and hold your elbows. Let your head hang from the root of the neck, which is between the shoulder blades. If it feels OK, work your neck a little: gently turn your head side to side or in a circle 2 or 3 times. Hold the position for 20 to 30 seconds. Then bring your hands onto your hips and SLOWLY straighten up.

Adaptations: Rest your hands just above your knees.
Can also be done while seated.

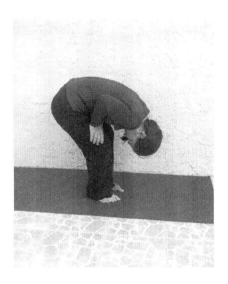 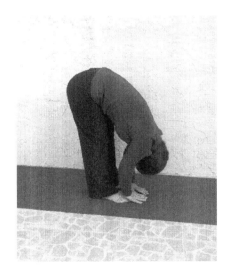

Your concept of yourself determines the world in which you live.
- Neville Goddard

Child Pose

A gentler version can be done in a chair. See "Seated Child Pose" below. Try both arm positions shown. One stretches the muscles along your spine, the other opens the shoulder blade area and relaxes your back.

Benefits: Calms the brain; relieves stress and fatigue. Relaxes your back muscles and stretches hips, thighs and torso.

Actions: Kneel on the floor or mat. Touch your big toes together and sit back by your heels. Separate your knees as wide apart as your hips. Rest your torso down between your thighs. Feel your ribcage expand and contract as you breathe. Relax in the pose for as long as you like.

Variations: (Photo 1) Rest your arms alongside you, palms up, and let your shoulders sink in front of the knees, if they will. Feel the shoulder blades widen across your back. You may prefer (Photo 2) reaching your arms out in front of you, palms down.

Adaptations: If sitting back by your heels is uncomfortable, place a folded blanket between your back thighs and calves.

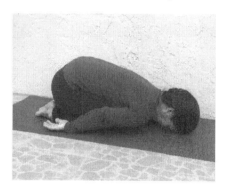 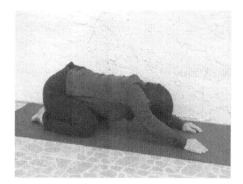

Seated Child Pose

There is no photo for this... Sitting at a table or desk, place one hand on top of the other, palms down, on the table in front of you. Rest your forehead there, and relax your neck, shoulders and back for a few slow, deep breaths. Then let your breath return to normal. Relax and breathe mindfully for at least 30 seconds.

Build Your Own Workout Sets

Use the charts on the following pages to make sets with various benefits. Choose from exercises in the Samples and Exercise Summary (Chapters 4, 5 and 6).

Here are 3 filled-in charts, as examples, followed by 6 blank charts (2 per page).

You could photocopy blank charts for making new sets, whenever you wish. (As you know, your brain likes new things.)

Enjoy growing your optimum mental fitness!

Brain-Building Workout Chart
(Sample 1)

Set Name _____*Recharge at my desk*_____
Brain Benefits ____*Energy, Clarity, Memory*_____
This Set Takes __3__ Minutes

Exercise (or Set) Name	Page #	Time	Notes
___Columns___	60	30 sec.	
___Thumb and Pinky	69	30 sec.	
___Trace the Wheel	70	30 sec.	
___Draw 8's with Eyes, Smiling	58	30 sec.	
___Mindful Breathing	82	1 min.	

Brain-Building Workout
(Sample 2)

Set Name ____*More Energy, Less Stress*_____
Brain Benefits __*Build & improve circuits, reduce stress*__
This Set Takes __4__ Minutes

Exercise	Page #	Time	Notes
Exhale!	*61*	*1 min.*	
8's and 0's	*66*	*30 sec.*	
Crossover Challenges	*53*	*1 min.*	*do #1 & 2*
Beach Ball Twist	*54*	*30 sec.*	
Seated Side Stretch	*68*	*30 sec.*	
Mindful Breathing	*82*	*30 sec.*	

Brain-Building Workout
(Sample 3)

Set Name ___ *Balance & Calm* _____
Brain Benefits __*Improve balancing skill, mental focus*__
This Set Takes __5_ Minutes

Exercise	Page #	Time	Notes
Deep breathing	*81*	*1 min*	
Mindful Walking	*84*	*2 min.*	
Balancing Circle	*74*	*30 sec*	
Tree Pose	*75*	*1 min*	*2x each side*
Energy Link	*85*	*1 min.*	*smile*

Brain-Building Workout

Set Name _____

Brain Benefits _____

This Set Takes ____ *Minutes*

Exercise	*Page #*	*Time*	*Notes*

Brain-Building Workout

Set Name _____

Brain Benefits _____

This Set Takes ____ *Minutes*

Exercise	*Page #*	*Time*	*Notes*

Brain-Building Workout

Set Name _____

Brain Benefits _____

This Set Takes _____ *Minutes*

Exercise	Page #	Time	Notes

Brain-Building Workout

Set Name _____

Brain Benefits _____

This Set Takes _____ *Minutes*

Exercise	Page #	Time	Notes

Brain-Building Workout

Set Name _____

Brain Benefits _____

This Set Takes _____ *Minutes*

Exercise	*Page #*	*Time*	*Notes*

Brain-Building Workout

Set Name _____

Brain Benefits _____

This Set Takes _____ *Minutes*

Exercise	*Page #*	*Time*	*Notes*

7

Mindful Meditation
to untangle the tangle...

"WHY DO WE MEDITATE?" Our retreat leader asked us, as we embarked on a week of mindfulness practice. "To untangle the tangle we create in the mind," he answered.

"Meditating is like slowing down an airplane propeller until you can actually see each blade," he said. When we slow the mind down, we notice every thought and feeling arising and passing away.

Our retreat leader was Bhante Rahula, a Theravada Buddhist monk. We were at Bhavana Society forest monastery and retreat center in West Virginia, where I've participated in several retreats, sometimes leading yoga sessions and serving as retreat coordinator.

Bhavana's founding Abbot is Bhante Gunaratana, author of *Mindfulness in Plain English*, a simple introduction to meditation.

"Bhavana" is a Pali word meaning "development" or "cultivation." I have been fortunate to study under "Bhante G", as many affectionately call him, and other excellent instructors at Bhavana.

Mindful Meditation, Defined

The word meditation comes from the Latin roots "medi" meaning "middle" and "tare" (pronounced 'tah-ray') meaning "ground". Hence, meditation means "middle ground." It benefits the brain and mind, as it synchronizes the hemispheres and reduces stress.

This practice is not religious. It is not about creating images in the mind, or blanking out the mind.

Mindfulness is *direct experience of the now*. It is awareness of each thought, sensation, and emotion.

In this practice, we notice our thoughts but do not grasp and ruminate over them. We let them go, and focus on the breath or other sensations, for present-moment awareness.

In the book, *10 Mindful Minutes*, Goldie Hawn describes it as:

"...accepting this awareness with openness and curiosity in a nonjudgmental way. It means focusing our attention on non-doing, a crucial skill in these distracted times." [1]

Brain Waves During Meditation

Electrical activity is always occurring in your brain. The type and location of electrical waves (delta, theta, alpha, and beta) are good indicators of brain activity.

A 2010 study found that meditating increases alpha and theta brain waves, associated with wakeful, relaxed attention. Study participants were experienced in Acem Meditation, a nondirective method developed in Norway. They were asked to rest with eyes closed for 20 minutes, and to meditate for another 20 minutes, in random order.

Their alpha and theta waves were more abundant during meditation than during relaxation. These waves originate from awareness that monitors inner experiences, the researchers noted.

"Here lies a significant difference between meditation and relaxing without any specific technique," said the lead researcher, Jim Lagopoulos, Ph.D.[2]

Meditation Builds the Brain

Mindfulness-Based Stress Reduction (MBSR) is a program developed by Dr. John Kabat-Zinn at the University of Massachusetts Medical Center. MBSR is now a widely-used mindfulness training program, aiding physical and psychological wellness.

Actual brain changes were observed in participants of an 8-week mindfulness-based stress reduction program. A study showed increased gray matter in brain regions involved in learning, memory, regulation of emotion, and self-awareness, as reported in the journal, *Psychiatry Research: Neuroimaging.*[3]

In another recent study, participants in a four-week mindfulness training showed increased efficiency of white matter, while other participants, in relaxation training, did not.

Researchers stated, "this dynamic pattern of white matter change involving the anterior cingulate cortex, a part of the brain network related to self-regulation, could provide a means for intervention to improve or prevent mental disorders." [4]

"It is important to view meditation not as a passive activity, but as an active, brain-stimulating exercise." - David Perlmutter, M.D.

Consistent practice of meditation increases the production of growth factor BDNF in your brain, according to Dr. Perlmutter. Mindful meditation develops a brain that is "not only more resistant to deterioration, but one that enables you to push the limits of day-to-day functionality," he explains.[5]

"Breath is the intersection of the body and mind." -*Thich Nhat Hanh*

Breath awareness is a good focal point for keeping the mind fully present. Brief instructions are given in the mindful breathing exercise on page 82, and there's a link to walking meditation instruction (including breath awareness) at the end of this chapter.

Without this fixed reference of breath-awareness, Bhante Gunaratana says, "you get lost, overcome by the ceaseless waves of change flowing round and round within the mind."[6]

The wandering mind can be compared to a wild elephant, as Bhante G describes in his book. As we meditate, the mind naturally wanders away from the breath and we keep gently bringing it back.

Taming the wild elephant

For centuries, elephants in Asia have played valuable roles in cultural ceremonies, logging and construction work. As a native of Sri Lanka, Bhante G has seen plenty of elephants. In *Mindfulness in Plain English, he writes:*

"Ancient Pali texts liken meditation to the process of taming a wild elephant. The procedure in those days was to tie a newly captured animal to a post with a good strong rope. When you do this, the elephant is not happy. He screams and tramples and pulls against the rope for days. Finally it sinks through his skull that he can't get away, and he settles down. At this point you can begin to feed him and to handle him with some measure of safety. Eventually you can dispense with the rope and post altogether and train your elephant for various tasks. Now you've got a tamed elephant that can be put to useful work.

In this analogy, the wild elephant is your wildly active mind, the rope is mindfulness, and the post is your object of meditation—your breathing. The tamed elephant which emerges from this process is a well-trained, concentrated mind that can then be used for the tough job of piercing the layers of illusion that obscure reality. Meditation tames the mind."[7]

Practicing Awareness

Any activity can be done as a mindful meditation. If you're new to it, you could try saying a few words silently to yourself as you practice. For example: while turning a doorknob, say to yourself, "turning, turning". As you open the door, say "opening, opening." Brushing your teeth, say "brushing, brushing." The words are not necessary; being fully present is what counts.

Seated Meditation

Fred Eppsteiner teaches for the Florida Community of Mindfulness. He reminds us to focus on the lower body as we begin a sitting session. Feeling legs and buttocks touching the seat keeps us grounded, and not caught up in the "thinking head," Eppsteiner says.

To enhance the centered feeling, some meditators have eyes slightly open and look toward the tip of the nose or other focal points. Some use "3rd Eye Gazing" described in Chapter 6. Placing the tip of the tongue on the roof of your mouth may also help. Some practitioners like to wear a half-smile. None of these techniques are required for a good meditation practice. The key is maintaining relaxed awareness in mind and body.

Mindfulness Training

Applications of MBSR in healthy aging, education, and the military are being studied by neuroscientists like Dr. Amishi Jha, Associate Professor of Psychology at the University of Miami.

In 2008, Dr. Jha teamed up with Dr. Elizabeth Stanley of Georgetown University in Washington, D.C., to offer mindfulness-based fitness training for soldiers. They wanted to see if mindful practices might prevent some of the mental health problems exhibited by many soldiers returning from Iraq.

The researchers recruited a civilian control group and two groups of Marines preparing for deployment to Iraq. All participants were tested for short-term memory skills, prior to just one group (of Marines) receiving an eight-week mindfulness training.

Only the mindful group showed improvements in short-term memory skills, on post-training tests.

Some of the "mindful" Marines continued practicing in Iraq, and reported more awareness of the warning signs of overstress, and more cooperative behavior within their teams.

"Mindful training exercises are showing promise as tools to build more attentive, less reactive brains," said Dr. Jha.[8]

For Children: A program called MindUP employs mindfulness training in school settings. Developed through the Hawn Foundation, established by Goldie Hawn, MindUp sessions help children understand where their emotions come from. They learn tools for reducing stress, sharpening concentration, and controlling how they respond to events in their world.[9]

Walking meditation instruction:
http://www.insightmeditationcenter.org/books-articles/articles/instructions-for-walking-meditation/

8

Best Brain Nutrition

BRAIN-FRIENDLY FOOD IS FOUND "in gardens, fields, orchards, rivers and seas. The less processed it is, the better," observes Dr. Paul Bendheim in *The Brain Training Revolution.*

Essential nutrients are more effective in their natural state, "as real food, rather than isolated, purified or synthesized as supplements in capsules or tablets," he adds.

Food industry wizards have become proficient at adding extracted nutrients to processed foods. Along with this trend, we have more obesity, heart disease, diabetes, and most recently, Alzheimer's disease, Dr. Bendheim explains.[1]

Take it from Popeye …

Leafy greens promote strong muscles and help your brain cells thrive. In the classic cartoon, Popeye the Sailor chugs a can of spinach whenever he needs to plump his biceps for amazing physical feats. His girlfriend is aptly named "Olive Oil."

Of course, spinach is healthier if eaten raw or slightly steamed, rather than overcooked and canned. And drizzling it with olive oil adds more brain benefits of healthy fat.

Spinach contains plenty of folate, a B-Vitamin that helps produce and maintain cells. The Vitamin B-6 in spinach increases your brain's serotonin and norepinephrine, which enhance energy and mood. It helps produce melatonin, to regulate your body clock.[2]

Deeply colored fruits and vegetables have high amounts of flavonoids, found in all plants. These are pigments which exert antioxidant activity to protect your brain from damage by free radicals. Purple foods like blueberries, grapes, plums, cranberries, acai, and eggplant are especially recommended.

Other good flavonoid sources are apples, peanuts, onions, red wine, tea and dark chocolate with no milk products in it.

For vibrant health, "Eat a variety of vegetables, fruits, raw nuts and seeds, and whole grains. Avoid heavily processed foods, animal products, added salt, and sugar. Aim to get 80 percent of your calories from carbohydrates, 10 percent from fat, and 10 percent from protein." This whole foods, plant-based diet is recommended by T. Colin Campbell, Ph.D., in *WHOLE: Rethinking the Science of Nutrition.*[3]

I am not pushing a totally vegetarian diet. Obviously, your brain can stay healthy if you eat fish, meats, eggs, and dairy products.

I do want to mention what statistics reveal: populations with mainly plant-based diets have less diseases than those regularly consuming meat and milk products. They also have healthier kidneys, bones and eyes.[4]

Healthy Fats

Your brain is composed of 60 percent fat, and having the right kinds of fats will help reduce your risk of mental disease, states Dr. Alan Logan in *The Brain Diet.*[5]

"If I had to pick only one dietary factor that could change your psychological condition, Omega-3s would be it," he writes.

Omega-3 and Omega-6 are "essential fats" – necessary for good health, but not produced by our bodies, so we must get them from foods. Some foods that contain good amounts of Omega fats are:

Oily fish, such as salmon, tuna, halibut, trout, sardines and herring. Vegetable sources of Omegas include nuts, seeds, avocados, beans, olives and vegetable oil.

Flax seed is high in Omega fats. You can put it in a coffee grinder and use it right away, while the nutrients are at their best. Or freeze the ground seed for up to two weeks. Try flax on top of oatmeal, or mixed in with various foods.

Walnuts. Just ¼ cup of walnuts has 2.3 grams of omega-3 fats. That's about 91% of the daily amount recommended by the U.S. Food and Drug Administration.[6]

Olive oil and other plant-based oils are rich in unsaturated fats.

Hummus (made from garbanzo beans) is a good source when it's made with sesame tahini, which has very high Omega-3 content.

Kale, Purslane and other greens are good sources of Omega 3 fats, calcium, iron and postassium. They can be added to a salad or served steamed, alone or with other veggies.

"Bad" Fats

You can reduce your risk of stroke and heart disease by limiting your intake of saturated and trans fats.

Meat and dairy products contain saturated fat, which increases your blood concentration of low-density lipoprotein (LDL), commonly called "bad" cholesterol. LDL increases your risk for heart disease and stroke.

Trans fats include margarine, shortening, or any "partially hydrogenated" fat or oil. They also increase LDL levels. Trans fats can be found in fast foods and processed baked goods such as chips, cookies and pies. Check the nutrition labels on packaged foods, for the amount of trans fats contained in them.

Coconut Oil and Cognitive Function

The University of South Florida is conducting a clinical trial of coconut oil for mild to moderate cases of Alzheimer's.

In these patients, some parts of the brain stop producing glucose, the main source of energy. MCT fats in coconut oil are converted by the liver into ketones, which are an alternate source of energy.

Ketones have been shown to recharge metabolic processes within the brain, "resulting in an almost immediate improvement in cognitive function," writes Sayer Ji, Founder of GreenMedInfo.com.

Dr. Mary Newport has documented such improvements in the book, *Alzheimer's Disease: What If There Was A Cure?* See Resources section.

All brains can benefit from consuming MCT fats—not just those with Alzheimer's. Sayer Ji suggests using it in place of vegetable oils, which are rancid and pro-inflammatory. "Or enjoy a delicious curry with coconut milk as a base. Because 25% of coconut milk is fat, and about 66% of that fat is MCT, you are still getting a healthy dose," he writes.[7] In addition, curry feeds your brain cells with its turmeric content. See "Spices for Your Brain", later in this chapter.

Enhancing Nutrients

When you have a little healthy fat with your vegetables, your body more easily absorbs the carotenoids (beta-carotene and lycopene) in them. These act as antioxidants to keep neurons healthy.

A recent study compared nutrient absorption in seven men and women after eating salads with varying levels of fat. They found only negligible amounts of carotenoids in their blood after eating a salad with fat-free dressing. Significantly more carotenoids appeared in their blood after eating salads with dressings containing fats.[8]

Calories Down, Memory Up

Research indicates that lower-calorie diets may benefit the brain.

In a 2009 study, a group of older adults showed a 20 percent improvement in verbal memory scores, after reducing their caloric intake by 30 percent for three months. Two other groups consumed their normal amount of calories during that time, and their memory scores did not change.[9]

In other studies, production of BDNF (the growth factor that enhances neurogenesis) rose dramatically in animals given 30 percent fewer calories in their diets, writes David Perlmutter, M.D., in *Power Up Your Brain.*

You're already sweet enough, right?

Eating less sugar, for many people, would simplify the cutting of calories, Dr. Perlmutter adds. The average American consumes too much refined sugar, which is linked to reduced BDNF levels and a corresponding reduction in memory function.[10]

Berries

Natural compounds in berries help with neuron signaling for clear thinking and motor control. Blueberries have an especially positive effect on memory skills, according to research conducted through the University of Cincinnati.

A group in their 70s with early memory decline showed significant improvement on learning and memory tests after consuming blueberry juice for two months.

Regular supplementation with blueberries may help offset degeneration of neurons, the researchers reported.[11]

Carbohydrates

Glucose, the form of sugar that powers your brain, is obtained through the carbohydrates ("carbs") you consume.

Avoid excess starches and refined carbs like white bread, potatoes, white rice, sweets, and sugary drinks. They cause spikes and dips in blood sugar as they digest quickly, and leave you feeling hungry again.

Complex carbs provide energy that lasts. These are found in whole grains, whole beans, and fresh vegetables (except for starchy ones, like potatoes), and some fruits, such as apples, plums, and cherries.

Check the glycemic levels. Foods with lower glycemic amounts slowly release glucose into your bloodstream. This gradual release helps minimize blood sugar swings and keep your brain energy balanced. You can find glycemic index lists in various books on nutrition, and at many websites.

The Franklin Institute shares information on nutrition and brain health, including a glycemic index, at:

http://www.fi.edu/learn/brain/carbs.html

Spices for Your Brain

Turmeric. Curcumin is the primary ingredient in the spice turmeric. It increases BDNF, and helps the brain with antioxidant, anti-inflammatory, antifungal and antibacterial properties, states David Perlmutter, M.D., in *Power Up Your Brain.*

In India, where turmeric is often used in curried recipes, the incidence of Alzheimer's is only 25 percent as high as in the United States. Enhanced BDNF production in the brains of those consuming turmeric is the most likely reason why they resist this brain disorder.[12]

Sage, oregano, and thyme have phytochemicals, which help preserve memory and cognitive function.[13]

Cinnamon is metabolized into sodium benzoate, which produces neurotrophic factors—"Miracle-Gro" proteins, like BDNF—in your brain. These factors stimulate the birth of neurons in the brain and strengthen the existing ones. Cinnamon has also been shown to reduce blood sugar levels in people with type II diabetes and reduce cholesterol by up to 25%, notes Gary Wenk, Ph.D., author of *Your Brain on Food.*[14]

Cheers For Chocolate

This delectable treat can be called "brain health food" as long as it's not loaded with milk and sugar. Chocolate contains flavonoids, which improve blood flow to the brain and heart, and protect your cells. Having moderate amounts of chocolate may boost cognitive performance.[15]

Dark chocolate, containing no milk, is best. *Nature Journal* reports that milk interferes with the absorption of antioxidants from chocolate and may negate its potential health benefits.[16]

Higher concentrations of cacao are said to have more flavonoids and bring more health benefits. Labels on some dark chocolate bars now clearly show the percentage of cacao in them.

You can develop a taste for bittersweet chocolate, if you gradually increase the percentage of cacao you choose.

Semi-sweet dark baking chocolate contains cocoa butter and some sugar but no dairy products. Cocoa butter is a natural fat, from cocoa beans. It is not hydrogenated, and has no trans fat. Its saturated fat is mostly stearic acid, shown to have no effect on blood cholesterol levels.[17]

Read labels before buying; many bittersweet or semi-sweet chocolates now contain little or no dairy products. Watch for casein and whey, which are derived from milk.

Red Wine, Grape Skins, Grape Juice, Peanuts

These contain significant amounts of resveratrol, an antioxidant which may have "neuroprotective properties" that reduce symptoms of Alzheimer's, ischemic stroke, Parkinson's, and epilepsy, according to the journal, *Biofactors.*[18]

Conflicting reports continue to surface about the value of resveratrol, and how much of it is present in various foods. To shed light on this, an article by Joe Keffer on *Livestrong.com* lists foods with resveratrol, and opinions on what it may do for brain health: http://www.livestrong.com/article/83831-sources-resveratrol/

What To Drink?

Water. It keeps the electrical energy humming in your brain. Water is vital for transporting nerve messages between brain cells. Get at least 64 ounces a day, and more if you are sweating from work or exercise. Dehydration can occur from excess salt or alcoholic beverages. If you're consuming them, drink extra water.

Fresh juices. Using a juice extractor provides nutrients of fresh fruit and veggies without having to consume the fiber, which takes time to digest. I recommend watering down your juice (whether it's homemade or not) to 2/3 juice and 1/3 water, especially if it's fruit juice, to avoid a spike in blood sugar level.

Smoothies. Blender-made with fresh veggies and fruit, smoothies are a great way to nourish your brain. See the green smoothie recipe at the close of this chapter.

Tea. It helps reduce the formation of plaques which cause a breakdown of communication between neurons, as occurs in Alzheimer's patients.

At the University of Newcastle upon Tyne, researchers found both green and black tea inhibit the enzymes associated with Alzheimer's Disease.

Green tea's inhibitive action outlasted that of black tea by six days in this study. The research team is working to develop a medicinal tea that might help Alzheimer's sufferers.[19]

Coffee. The caffeine in coffee helps with alertness and memory, by boosting circulation in key areas of the brain. It increases the feel-good chemicals in the brain. There are pros and cons to consuming caffeine.

Moderate coffee consumption can appreciably lower the risk of Alzheimer's Disease or delay its onset, say researchers at the University of South Florida.[20]

How Caffeine Revs Us Up

Many of us enjoy tea or coffee in the morning. Some folks I know say they aren't fully awake until their caffeine kicks in. How does this magical substance affect brain chemicals?

In your brain, caffeine mimics a chemical called adenosine, which is produced by neurons as they fire. Your nervous system monitors adenosine levels through receptors. When enough receptors have been activated by adenosine, "your nervous system pays off the tab by putting you to sleep," writes David DiSalvo.

By mimicking adenosine, caffeine blocks its receptors and disrupts its monitoring by the nervous system. Then the neurotransmitters dopamine and glutamate, "are freer to do their stimulating work," DiSalvo explains. "In other words, it's not the caffeine that's doing the stimulating. Instead, it's keeping the doors blocked while the real party animals of the brain do what they love to do." [21]

Caffeine drinkers who depend on that morning boost may have symptoms like headaches or sleepiness for a few days, if they stop having caffeine.

Caffeine is abundant in chocolate, coffee, tea, many soft drinks, and energy drinks. Moderating or eliminating caffeine can help our brains stay well balanced.

What Not To Drink

Sugary drinks. *They* cause an over-abundance of glucose in your blood, which results in lower insulin levels in your brain. Insulin is needed for your neurons to absorb glucose and do their jobs well.

Too much alcohol. A moderate intake of alcoholic beverages may have health benefits for most people. But alcohol can cause dehydration. As a diuretic, it causes you to urinate more often, ultimately expelling more liquid than you take in.

As you know, heavy drinking may fuel depression/anxiety, addiction, and a host of related issues. Excess alcohol depletes energy, inhibits new brain cell growth, and impairs thought processes.

Too much caffeine. It may cause "the jitters" or an upset stomach. It blocks adenosine receptors and affects your nervous system, as previously mentioned.

Cooking methods make a difference

Steaming, boiling and poaching methods use lower temperatures than frying, baking or grilling. When exposed to very high temperatures, foods produce more chemical end-products that cause inflammation and oxidative stress.

Grains Affect Brains

Intolerance or sensitivity to glutens (found in wheat and other grains) causes serious digestive problems. Science has recently revealed that glutens affect the brain, as well as the digestive system.

Mayo Clinic researchers uncovered a link between dementia and celiac disease, a digestive condition caused by gluten intolerance.

Joseph Murray, M.D., a study investigator, suggests finding and treating celiac disease early can prevent symptoms in digestive and brain functions.

For celiac disease patients who have shown cognitive decline, following a gluten-free diet may help reduce their symptoms.[22]

Florida neurologist David Perlmutter, M.D., has seen brain functions improve in affected patients who removed glutens from their diets. "Gluten sensitivity is one of the few truly treatable factors in some dementia cases," he says. "And it's terribly under-recognized."

"Everyone should be concerned about what modern wheat could be doing, not just to their brain, but to their entire physiology," he adds.[23]

Grain Brain, Dr. Perlmutter's most recent book, provides ground-breaking facts on how wheat and other grains impact brain function.

I also recommend *The Dark Side of Wheat,* by Sayer Ji. It can be found at http://www.greenmedinfo.com as noted in the Resources.

Consult with a health professional about nutritional supplements or any major changes to your diet.

Treat your brain to a delicious *Green Smoothie!*
What? Combine greens with fruit? Yes.

Victoria Boutenko, author of *Green Smoothie Revolution,* says the fiber in green leaves helps slow the absorption of natural sugars in fruit, making it helpful in smoothies. Plus, the fruit helps the greens go down!

Boutenko relates what sparked her "green smoothie revolution."

"Green leaves don't have starch, while vegetables such as carrots, beets, broccoli, etc., contain a lot of starch. Starchy vegetables combined with fruit may cause bloating. That discovery marked the beginning...I peeled bananas and blended them with green kale. With trepidation, I opened the lid of the blender and it smelled great. I tasted this super green drink and it tasted exactly like a banana smoothie. I was able to trick my body...I ecstatically enjoyed the greens for the first time in my life! [24]

"Parsley Passion"
 - Sergei Boutenko

1 bunch fresh parsley
1 cucumber, peeled
1 Fuji apple
1 ripe banana
1 to 2 cups water
Mix all in blender and enjoy.

Find awesome smoothie and soup recipes in the book, *The Green Smoothie Revolution,* and online at:
http://www.rawfamily.com/recipes

9

Brains Love Laughing!

We do not laugh because we are happy.
We are happy because we laugh.
-William James

IT'S 8:00 ON A BREEZY MORNING at Fort Myers Beach, Florida. Towels and beach mats are spread on the sand, as over a dozen people gather and stand in a circle. They smile and make eye contact.

"Ho-ho, ha-ha-ha!" The group starts cheering over and over, clapping with the beat. Instructor Meg Scott guides them in stretching, breathing, and silly-making gestures.

Soon there are giggles, then hearty guffaws. Arms up high, they shout, "Very good, very good—Yay!" After the funny exercises, they have stretching and several minutes of deep relaxation.

This Laughter Yoga workout started in Mumbai, India, in 1995. Dr. Madan Kataria led the first group—of just five people—in "laughing for no reason." Thousands of such groups now meet in over 65 countries.[1]

"It feels artificial at first, but then it gets to your funny bone, and you're really laughing," said Lisa Gentile, a participant at Fort Myers Beach. "It starts my day on a positive note."

Loma Linda University studies have shown how laughter diffuses tension by decreasing your levels of cortisol and epinephrine, the "stress chemicals." Dr. Lee Berk and his colleagues reported positive effects of humor on the immune system. It increases antibodies and helps destroy tumor cells.

Their findings show that repetitious "mirthful laughter" causes the body to respond in a way similar to moderate physical exercise.[2]

"Our everyday behaviors and emotions affect our bodies in many ways," Dr. Berk explains. "As the old biblical wisdom states, it may indeed be true that laughter is a good medicine."

A dose of humor

Smiling and laughing elevate your brain's level of dopamine, a neurotransmitter that triggers pleasure and improves attention and motivation. A Stanford University research team examined the brains of study participants who looked at funny cartoons, and found measurable activation in their limbic systems, where the brain regulates dopamine. In a 2003 issue of *Neuron Journal,* the researchers noted that humor enhances mood, motivation and concentration.[3]

Try an experiment with me...As you read the rest of this chapter (minus the exercises) keep a big smile on your face. Yes, curl up the corners of your mouth, show your teeth, and hold that smile!

"Smiling on purpose" is highly recommended by Cliff Kuhn, M.D., for mind/brain health. Since smiling boosts your mood and energy level, Dr. Kuhn prescribes it for hundreds of depressed patients. He says, "Those willing to practice it *always report* mood elevation and a reduction in symptoms—almost instantly!"

"These benefits kick in, even if you wear a fake smile!" he adds.[4]

Television networks have featured the benefits of "laughing on purpose." In 2006, Dr. Sanjay Gupta discussed laughter in a CNN series, *"Happiness and your Health."* [5] Dr. Gupta also promoted "fake laughter for a long life" in an interview by Conan O'Brien on TBS.[6]

Back in India, Dr. Kataria's laughter club grew fast and caught the attention of Mumbai's media, which marveled at "how (otherwise sane) adults can have such fun behaving like idiots at 7 a.m. in a public park."[7]

Two years later, Dr. Kataria quit his medical practice and began working full time on teaching and promoting Laughter Yoga.

Around the same time, Dr. Patch Adams was spreading mirth in hospital wards, using laughter to help people heal. Actor Robin Williams starred in the 1998 film, "Patch Adams," based on the doctor's life and work.

Did you Try the Experiment?

If you tried "holding a smile" as you were reading, I wonder how you're feeling now? Do you notice any changes in your body/mind?

"Laughter changes your mood within minutes," says Meg Scott, certified Laughter Leader at Fort Myers Beach. "The more you laugh and smile, the more positive your outlook becomes."

Want to find a laughter group near you? See Resources, for ideas.

10

Remedy for Stress

YOUR BODY RESPONDS TO DANGER by producing stress hormones (cortisol and adrenaline) to increase the heart rate and blood pressure while inhibiting digestion. Extra blood flows quickly toward your extremities, priming your muscles to "fight or flee." You've probably heard or read about this "fight or flight" response.

Problem: Chronic Stress. Today's humans secrete stress hormones constantly, in response to psychological pressures of everyday life, says Dr. Robert Sapolsky, a Stanford Neurobiologist. Our highly-evolved intelligence can work against us (creating needless worries) if we're not careful.

Chronic stress diminishes brain cells and the circuits involved in memory and learning. "It's becoming clear that in the hippocampus, the part of the brain most susceptible to stress hormones, you see atrophy in people with post-traumatic stress disorder and major depression," he observes.

Excess cortisol is related to weight gain; it disrupts fat distribution and may cause a "spare tire" around the middle.

Stress overload accelerates chromosome aging, Sapolsky adds. People with stressful lives "grow old" faster than those with less stress.[1]

Solution: Relax. It may seem too simple, but since the 1970's, Dr. Herbert Benson has been sharing his helpful technique, "Eliciting the Relaxation Response", described below.

Herbert Benson, M.D., is Associate Professor of Medicine and Founder of the Mind-Body Medical Institute at Harvard University. His 1976 classic book, *The Relaxation Response,* describes how endorphins (produced through relaxation) counteract stress hormones and reduce tension.

How To Elicit the Relaxation Response

1) Be in a comfortable, quiet space; 2) Close your eyes; 3) deeply relax all your muscles, starting with your feet and progressing up to your face. Keep them relaxed. 4) Breathe naturally, with awareness. Silently repeat the word "one" each time you exhale (or use another word or sound that carries little meaning, to avoid distracting your mind from relaxing). 5) Continue for 10 to 20 minutes, then slowly return to normal activities. Distracting thoughts will occur during the process, but keep bringing your mind back to the breath and the word you are repeating.[2]

Dr. Benson notes that deep relaxation comes easily with regular practice. Learn more about this technique and its benefits at the website: http://www.relaxationresponse.org Click on "How to Elicit the Relaxation Response, Step by Step."

If you attend a yoga class, it will probably include relaxation at the end. It helps to be guided into deep rest by an instructor. Yoga relaxation pose is translated as "Savasana" in Sanskrit, meaning "dissolving pose."☺

Guided relaxation recordings are available online and via CDs and DVDs. A few examples are listed in the Resources section.

11

Making New Grooves

"We choose and sculpt how our ever-changing minds will work."
– Michael Merzenich, Ph.D.

IN JULY OF 2009, I EXPERIENCED the worst tragedy of my life. My brother Paul died by suicide. He was 58.

Paul was my only brother, and I thankfully still have my only sister, Rita. When we were kids, my "big brother" Paul was always looking out for me. He was well-liked among neighbors, co-workers and friends, and gave plenty of attention to his children as they were growing up.

Years passed, and habits like alcohol abuse and financial negligence crept into Paul's world. With debts, depression, and two divorces, his low self-esteem fueled a downward spiral.

I, too, have suffered with low self-esteem and a former habit of heavy drinking. Paul and I both developed some deep insecurities, and I can relate to what was happening inside him.

The Path of Least Resistance
When you think and act, energy messages travel along circuits in your brain. When a thought or action is repeated over and over, certain circuits are strengthened. These are like "grooves" set in place by habit-patterns.

In scientific terms, repetition creates thicker myelin around nerve fibers, boosting a circuit's efficiency, as observed by John Ratey, M.D., mentioned in Chapter 2.

Neuroscientist / artist Greg Dunn creates images by blowing ink across paper. It spreads out along paths of least resistance, the way neurons grow, he says.[1]

The phrase "neurons that fire together, wire together" describes the reinforcing of brain circuits. Some stroke victims have rewired their circuits to regain the use of affected limbs, noted in Chapter 1. And practicing meditation creates brain changes, mentioned in Chapter 7.

Chronic pain also affects neural circuits. Frequent pain may create a "negative feedback loop" resulting in more pain, with emotional reactions, possibly leading to anxiety and depression.

But the good news: 1) Studies show that when chronic pain is successfully treated, brain effects can be reversed. 2) Mind-body practices (such as focusing attention) may reduce chronic pain.[2]

It's not easy to "make new grooves" in the brain, but it can be done, as discussed later in this chapter.

Brain-Driven Behavior

Uncontrolled behaviors based in addiction and obsession are driven mostly by brain activity. They occur "when the brain hijacks your will and causes you to act in ways that are unhelpful or downright destructive," explains Daniel Amen, M.D., in *Making a Good Brain Great.*[3]

Suicide, the sad culmination of negative, brain-driven thinking, is the tenth leading cause of adult deaths in the United States.[4]

Obsessive-compulsive disorder (OCD) is a medical condition involving brain-driven behavior. The person cannot shake an obsessive thought, and "must" act on it.

In addictions, brain actvity compels the person to keep relying on "the drug", which could be gambling, impulsive shopping, sex, food, controlling others, alcohol/drugs, or raging fits of anger. Have I left out any destructive addictions? You might think of more.

Brain scans at Dr. Amen's clinics have shown activity that's either too low or too high in patients with drug abuse issues.

"If the brain is overactive, alcohol or painkillers help abusers slow it down. If it's underactive, they may use cocaine or other stimulants to speed up the action," observes Dr. Amen.

Over 200 violent convicted felons have undergone brain scans at Amen clinics. "The dysfunction I saw was often dramatic," he writes.[5]

Will-driven behavior

Constructive behavior supports balanced living. It reflects a sense of meaning and purpose, and fosters healthy relationships. It helps us set and reach goals, and adjust them, if necessary.

This "will-driven behavior" is what most people exhibit in daily life. But when chemical imbalances, fears, or addictions are strong, the brain's activity can take over and "negatively drive" our thoughts and actions.

Do we all have the same level of free will? If the brain directs behavior and free will, and brain function is impaired, then we do not, Dr. Amen explains. "A person with a very healthy brain has nearly 100 percent free will. A patient with OCD or addiction has significantly less, and a person with late Alzheimer's disease has virtually none." [6]

Brains and Addiction

In many cases, doctor-prescribed drugs help relieve depression, anxiety or obsessive patterns by balancing brain chemistry. But what happens in the brain when relying on a drug (including alcohol or any addictive behavior) overrules a person's "free will"?

Your brain's limbic system contains the "reward circuit" which allows you to feel pleasure. It is activated through eating, sex, exercise, and creative outlets such as music or art. The reward circuit is also stimulated by alcohol/drugs, and habits like gambling. Dopamine and other "pleasure" chemicals in the brain are released through all these activities.

Over-stimulation of the reward circuit occurs in addictions (especially with alcohol/drugs). This creates a euphoria which teaches the person to repeat the behavior. It may become a refuge when they're stressed or need a lift.

The "tolerance effect" occurs as a brain responds to surges of dopamine, and other neurotransmitters involved in pleasure, by producing lower amounts of them, or reducing their receptors. As addiction progresses, larger amounts of the drug are needed to get a pleasure fix.

Addiction erodes a person's self-control and ability to make sound decisions, as the brain's energy follows the "path of least resistance" to the drug or behavior involved.

Grooves That Improve

The rest of this chapter offers ideas and encouragement for replacing destructive habits with fresh, enlivening ones.

An "Attitude of Gratitude"

A friend of mine lost her only child—a 14-year-old girl—in a car accident. Of course, Laura was devastated. Life felt dark and meaningless to her, long after her daughter died.

Then Laura told me she has a new habit: each night she thinks of three things she's thankful for, as she's drifting off to sleep. This helps to ease some of the sorrow, and keep her mind going in the right direction, she said.

Research has shown the benefits of focusing on what's going well. In a recent study, those who kept "gratitude journals" felt better about their lives, compared to those who wrote about problems or neutral events. The "thankful" subjects wrote each week in their journals. They were exercising more regularly, reporting less illness and more optimism about the coming week and their lives as a whole.[7]

Shedding Unwanted Habits

Whether it's a pesky issue like interrupting others when they're speaking, or a major obsession like washing hands fifity times a day, we can curb negative cycles of thinking and behaving. Here's an example:

After brief intensive cognitive-behavioral treatment at the University of California, San Diego, OCD patients had robust clinical improvements and changes in brain acivity, wrote Sanjaya Saxena, M.D., lead author in the 2008 study.

Brain scans of these patients showed increased activity in a region involved in reappraisal and suppression of negative emotions: the right dorsal anterior cingulate cortex. Activity in this region directly correlated with the degree of improvement in their symptoms.[8]

Keys to Changing Habits

~ *Self-Awareness: What Need Does This Habit Serve?* It helps to know the "why" behind a destructive pattern. In my case, alcohol helped me relax and escape worries about financial or relationship problems (which, of course, were both related to my drinking habit).

When I realized that relaxing, feeling comforted and secure are normal needs—and that I can fill them through life-giving activities like meditation, exercise, and laughing with friends—I more easily made the switch from drinking to living well.

~ *Filling the vacuum* with things we enjoy: Instead of going for a drink after work with friends, I cultivated friendships at the gym, took a writing class, joined a volunteer project...you get the idea!

~ *Nutrition Plays a Role* in alcohol, drug or food addictions. Keeping blood sugar in balance is essential, and a whole foods diet is recommended. Of course, it's best to discuss dietary changes with your doctor. Nutrition for recovery is discussed at the web page http://ezinearticles.com/515646

~ *Social support and daily exercise* are essential, in my opinion, for "making new grooves" and kicking harmful habits.

Getting High Naturally

You probably don't need this reminder, but I hope you'll share it with loved ones, as they conquer drinking, pills, or smoking habits.

Many activities give a natural "pleasure fix" and help us relax. *Music* stimulates the limbic region, evoking memories and emotions, as mentioned in Chapter 12. Playing instruments or listening to music can relieve stress and energize your body and mind. ***Exercise, smiling and laughing*** always result in mood enhancement. With a "natural high", there's no hangover the next morning...well, maybe a lingering smile. As the old saying goes, "Get high on life!"

Releasing old stories with new therapies

The brain sometimes needs help making new patterns, in persons who have suffered traumas or abuse. The natural instinct to protect oneself is strong, and victims may remain on emotional "high alert" without knowing it. They have difficulty trusting others; their relationships suffer, and self confidence is low.

Two new therapies involving brain activity have shown some promise as effective tools for change:

Eye Movement Therapy:

Using eye movements for brain activation, EMDR (Eye Movement Desensitization and Reprocessing) may assist in releasing traumatic memories. The patient follows a process of removing emotional charges about a past experience, while making specified eye movements.

Soldiers and others with severe traumatic memories have participated in trials of EMDR, with positive results. In some cases of PTSD (Post Traumatic Stress Disorder), EMDR was shown more helpful than "talk-it-out" psychotherapy.[9]

Emotional Freedom Technique:

Shown to alleviate lingering anxiety from traumas, Emotional Freedom Technique (EFT) involves tapping specific points on the body. Scientists speculate this helps by decreasing arousal of the limbic (emotional) system and other brain areas involved in "fight or flight" response. The tapping points connect to energy pathways identified in Traditional Chinese Medicine.

For soldiers having symptoms of PTSD, treatment with EFT was the focus of a recent study. Six sessions resulted in significant drops in participants' levels of anxiety, depression, and overall distress. Researchers state that "delivering EFT to returning vets may be an effective method for reducing this entire group of co-occurring psychological traumas."[10]

Knowledge Is Power

Understanding brain-driven behavior helps us cope with a loved-one's (or our own) destructive choices. Knowing how brain patterns develop, and how unhealthy thoughts and habits can spiral out of control, makes it easier to forgive and heal.

12

So Much More

WE HAVE AN ABUNDANCE OF ways to benefit our brains. This chapter covers some, and I know you can think of more.

Move Fast! Aerobic Exercise

Regular exercise is the best way to keep your brain healthy. It works better than intellectual activity, nutrition or medications, says Mayo Clinic director of Alzheimer's research, Dr. Ronald Petersen.

Aerobic exercise increases your brain's BDNF, the nerve growth factor mentioned in Chapter 1.

The exercises in this book promote full brain activation, but they are not aerobic workouts, which raise your heart rate and increase oxygen intake.

Elevating your heart rate for at least 20 minutes, 3 or more times a week, reduces your risk of mental decline.[1]

Any rhythmic activity that uses large muscle groups is considered aerobic in nature. Examples are: walking, running, dancing, swimming, and bicycling.

The Proceedings of the National Academy of Sciences reported that older adults who walked for 40 minutes, three times a week for a year, had growth in the hippocampus and improvements in memory.

The researchers noted a correlation between the larger hippocampus and greater serum levels of BDNF.[2]

Your brain's vitality gets a boost with voluntary exercise, which "enhances brain performance and is directly associated with increased production of BDNF," observes Dr. Perlmutter in *Power Up Your Brain*.

By exercising, "even to a relatively moderate degree, you can actively take control of your mental destiny."[3]

People with limited mobility can easily do light aerobic workouts, such as chair exercise. Many fitness centers now offer gentle classes.

Strength Training

Resistance training with weights can help improve memory, attention, problem solving, and decision-making, according to Pascale Michelon, Ph.D., author of *Max Your Memory*.

A group of women with probable mild cognitive impairment (MCI) participated in a study, working out with weights twice a week, for six months. The women took cognitive skills tests before starting weight training, and showed measurable improvements on follow-up tests after the training period.[4]

Brain scans showed increased blood flow to areas associated with the improved cognitive performance.

Evidently, a short period of time (six months) of resistance training can benefit people who are already suffering from cognitive impairment, writes Dr. Michelon.[5]

Strength training can be done using weight machines, free weights (barbells and dumbbells), resistance tubing (which provides resistance when stretched), and your own body weight (pushups, pull-ups, abdominal work and leg squats).

How much is needed? For most people, two to three sessions a week, lasting 20 to 30 minutes are sufficient. Fitness experts recommend doing resistance training every other day, interspersed with aerobic workouts.

Check with your doctor and perhaps a fitness trainer to discuss the type of weight training that suits your needs.

The Centers for Disease Control has a comprehensive guide to strength training: http://www.cdc.gov/physicalactivity/growingstronger

Learn and Grow

Activities requiring concentration are great for the brain. Practicing a new language or computer program, dance steps, yoga, or any skill gets the mind to focus, as neural circuits activate. Playing a musical instrument, gardening, creative writing, bird-watching, or reading about interesting topics are ways to keep nerve messages moving.

"Just doing the old dance steps you already know won't help your brain's motor cortex stay in shape," writes Norman Doidge, M.D. "To keep the mind alive requires learning something truly new, with intense focus."[6]

Puzzles, Games, Neurobics

Crosswords and Sudoku (Japanese number puzzles) are well-known aids in keeping brains spry. And since neurogenesis started getting more attention in the media, new tools for building brains have appeared in books, magazines, DVD's, and online.

You can search library catalogs or the internet, under brain games, brain puzzles, or brain fitness. On the web, you'll be amazed at the mountain of sites that pop up.

One called "Games for the Brain" has chess, checkers, and many other games to keep you sharp, at: http://www.gamesforthebrain.com That's one example of hundreds of such websites.

More active games for your brain are table tennis (ping pong), foosball, air hockey, and others involving eye-hand coordination, fast movements and decision-making. My sister Rita taught me the fast-moving card game called Spit; also called Slam or Speed. Although we now live 3,000 miles apart, I shall challenge Rita to a Spit championship, next time we visit! (So I'd better practice up, because she's quick.) Learn about the game of Spit at this site: http://boardgames.about.com/od/spit/a/spit_rules.htm.

If you like puzzles, I recommend a book that challenges many cognitive functions: *The Playful Brain.* For the variety of challenges in this book, Dr. Richard Restak described various brain functions that decline with age unless we work to keep them engaged. Scott Kim designed puzzles to work the brain areas involved in each of those functions, including: concentration, memory, fine motor skills, visual observation, logic, numbers, vocabulary, visual-spatial thinking, imagination, and creativity." [7] *Whew!* A three-pound brain manages so many functions!

"Neurobics" are activities that engage different parts of the brain in familiar tasks. Try getting dressed with your eyes closed to activate your sense of touch. Take a different route, driving home or walking the dog. Try eating, writing, or opening doors with your non-dominant hand, to strengthen pathways in the side of your brain that is less used. See "Expressing With Your Other Hand" exercise in Chapter 6.

Neurobics are featured in the book, *Keep Your Brain Alive*, by Lawrence Katz, Ph.D., and Manning Rubin.[8]

The Power of Music

You know the feeling: as you recognize a song you really like, your body responds with a smile, or waves of nostalgia.

Rhythm, dance and song have always been part of human civilization. Music brings us together in celebrations and ceremonies; greatly enhancing the "atmosphere" and affecting our moods.

Several parts of your brain respond and work together as you react to music, said neuroscientist Valorie Salimpoor. Your favorite music increases activity in the nucleus accumbens, causing your dopamine level to rise.[9] Other brain regions help you remember the words of a song and keep time with the beat.

Playing a musical instrument helps you build and maintain neural circuits, as both hands are involved.

Drum circles and traditional Native dances are ways to celebrate culture and maintain social connections. I enjoyed a performance by Alaska Native dancers from a remote village. "This is how we come together and stay active in our long winters," the group leader said.

Going out to enjoy live music gives you the added brain benefit of socializing, and perhaps you'd like to *dance!*

Dancing Brains

With coordinated movements, balance, memory and rhythm involved in dancing, your brain gets a great workout. New synapses are sprouting forth as your neural circuits are busy the entire time, and there's the fun and social aspect, too. Most people are smiling while dancing; how about you?

Drink little or no alcohol before dancing. Inebriation destroys the benefits!

A Playlist For Your Brain

As you know, listening to music can help you sleep, cheer you up, calm you down, or enhance your workout. Now there's a book explaining the science behind it.

Your Playlist Can Change Your Life is written by three psychologists, including Galina Mindlin, Ph.D.,psychiatry professor at Columbia University, and founder of Brain Music Therapy.

It helps to record songs into a player, in the order you choose (a playlist), the authors explain. iPods and other gadgets work well for making personal playlists, but if you don't have them, you can still select music to benefit your brain.[10]

Your favorite music can aid memory and alertness while enhancing energy and mood. So, fire up your iPod, arrange your albums, and fix your radio settings for a happy brain, mind and body.

Sleep

Your brain consolidates new information to memory while you're asleep. In recent studies, people who had slept after learning a task did better on remembering what they had learned.

Quality Z-time also keeps you mentally sharp. If you lose too much sleep, your stress hormone levels increase, making it harder to concentrate, according to Harvard Women's Health Watch.[11]

Most people function best with an average of 7 hours of sleep each night. If you're having trouble relaxing, you might try some of the "Refresher" exercises in this book. And regular aerobic exercise, even low impact, aids in getting restful sleep.

Oxygen!

Your brain uses about three times as much oxygen as your muscles use, so it's essential to keep the oxygen flowing upstairs.

Bringing attention to your breath is one key to getting enough oxygen, says Yoga instructor Erika Cooper, Founder of Elements Yoga in Bonita Springs, Florida.

"It's easy to underestimate the breath, considering it's an automatic function of our bodies. However, when you bring your attention to your breath, you can start to breathe deeply and fully, with awareness. The maximum exchange of oxygen occurs in the lower lungs but, most of the time, because of our posture and regular breathing habits, not much air seems to get down there," Erika explains.

The three-part breath exercise in this book allows you to get a full, deep breath. Or just try placing both hands on your belly, and consciously expanding it outward on the inhale, and drawing it back in on the exhale. Notice your hands moving with the breath.

"As more oxygen reaches your brain and body tissues, you have more energy, better digestion, and fewer headaches, all proven benefits of breathing deeply and fully," Erika adds.[12]

Oxygen Therapy

Studies have shown hyperbaric oxygen (HBO) therapy can inhibit some of the damaging effects of a stroke, if it's caught in time. In HBO therapy, the patient is in a room or a chamber where the air pressure is raised up to three times higher than normal. Their lungs can then gather three times as much oxygen, to promote healing.

This therapy has been shown to reduce migraine headache pain and prevent cluster headaches by lowering pressure within the cranium. It has accelerated neurological recovery after spinal cord injuries, and helped heal serious wounds and infections.

The National Institutes of Health has reported promising results with HBO therapy for stroke, atherosclerosis, cerebral palsy, headache and brain and spinal cord injury.[13]

Regarding oxygen treatment for stroke, Dr. Perlmutter said, "It is always much more helpful to treat patients as soon after the event as possible. Unfortunately, many patients remain hospitalized in the early post-stroke period and generally this precludes hyperbaric therapy, as most hospitals do not embrace the utility of this profoundly effective therapy."[14]

Aroma and the Brain

Does the smell of coffee, apple pie, cinnamon, or lemon bring forth good feelings in you? The brain's limbic (emotional) system is directly connected with smell receptors in your nostrils, which explains how a scent can conjure specific memories and associations.

The University of Maryland Medical Center reports that several essential oils are shown helpful in relieving anxiety, stress, and depression: lavender, rose, orange, bergamot, lemon, and sandalwood.[15]

Scents are used in aromatherapy—sometimes along with a massage treatment. Essential oils derived from plants produce certain effects, i.e., basil may help increase mental clarity and concentration, while lavender and chamomile have a calming effect.

At the Medical University of Vienna, Austria, a 2005 study found that scents are capable of altering emotional states. Researchers noted lavender and orange scents reduced anxiety and improved mood in patients waiting for dental treatment.[16]

For Alzheimer's patients, a few studies have noted reduced anxiety after using aromatherapy; however, more objective clinical research is needed to confirm the benefits of this treatment.

Your Brain In Love

A well-functioning brain is necessary for satisfying relationships of all kinds. Your brain dictates your perceptions and attitudes; it makes decisions on how to interact with others—what to say and do—all the time. If the brain works well, relationships go well.

Good relationships bring more joy and less stress; you smile and laugh often, and your brain gets these benefits.

Sexual relations are best in the context of a committed, loving relationship. I share this bias with Dr. Daniel Amen, as he explains it in his book, *The Brain In Love.*

"Your brain's health determines how well you do as a partner and a parent. It helps you be enthusiastic in the bedroom, or drains you of desire and passion," writes Dr. Amen.[17]

Your brains help you and your partner achieve wonderful orgasms, which in turn are great for your brains. Pleasure chemicals such as dopamine are released during orgasm. They enhance energy, mood, and mental clarity.

In essence, a good sexual relationship is about your state of mind, and brain.

Social Interactions

Enjoying good company helps you stay mentally alert and focused, as you engage in conversations and activities. You learn more and laugh more by being involved with others.

Seek discussions that spark your interest and rev up your brain circuits. Being in a club or activity group provides social interaction while doing something you enjoy. Volunteer work, book studies, bridge clubs, hiking groups and churches are ways of gathering for meaningful interactions. Exercise and meditation groups abound; you can even find them now in very small towns.

Nature and your Neurons

Here is your final exercise instruction in this book:

Engage with nature. Leave your cares behind; drop your "do-list" and enjoy being outdoors. Let Mother Nature feed your neurons.

"Mindful engagement with nature" is a simple, inexpensive way to clear the brain fog of daily hassles or cyber-info-overload, writes Dr. Eva Selhub, co-author (with John Wiley) of *Your Brain, On Nature.*

"Spending time walking or contemplating in a forest (compared to an urban setting), is associated with lower levels of cortisol and other physiological markers of stress," she explains.[18]

Nature walks provide fresh oxygen, better circulation and a retreat from the daily routine. Your brain appreciates it.

Epilogue

This is an exciting time to be alive! Intriguing details about brain plasticity are still being uncovered, with all corners of society showing an eager interest in them.

In education, sports, healthy aging, and mind-body wellness programs, brain fitness has become a buzz-word. Opportunities for growth abound for people (like yourself) focused on vibrant, meaningful living.

Earlier this year, President Obama announced a new program for researching brain cell functions, to better understand how the mind works, and hopefully find new ways to treat and prevent brain disorders.

Many things you're already doing stimulate neurons to grow and improve their connections. Just taking a walk builds the brain! Nutritious food, good social interactions, creative outlets like music and art, fresh air and exercise—all contribute to cognitive fitness.

You have the materials: a healthy brain and body, a determined mind, and ever-increasing knowledge. As you use the tools in this book, be ready for pleasant surprises. Your life will reflect the positive changes in your new best friend—the brain.

Comments about this book are welcome through emails. Send to: *info@preserveyourbrain.com*

Visit the website: http://www.preserveyourbrain.com

Resources & Reading

Find a brain-building seminar, fitness class, laughter group, etc., in:

Facilities, such as hospital wellness centers, education programs, fitness clubs, recreation and senior centers, yoga studios.
Newspapers: community calendars in print and online editions.
Natural health magazines, free in many health food stores, libraries, and natural health centers.
Libraries often have free community publications with event listings, as well as brain fitness books and audiovisual materials.

Books:
~ *SPARK: The Revolutionary New Science of Exercise and the Brain.* John Ratey, M.D. Little, Brown and Company, 2013
~ *Magnificent Mind At Any Age: Natural Ways to Unleash Your Brain's Maximum Potential.* Daniel G. Amen, M.D. Three Rivers Press, 2009
~ *The Brain That Changes Itself.* Norman Doidge, M.D. Penguin, 2007
~ *The Playful Brain: The Surprising Science of How Puzzles Improve Your Mind.* Richard Restak, M.D., and Scott Kim. Penguin Group, 2010
~ *Smart Moves: Why Learning Is Not All In Your Head.* Carla Hannaford, Ph.D. Great River Books, 2005
~ *Keep Your Brain Alive* (Neurobic exercises). Lawrence Katz, Ph.D and Manning Ruben. Workman Publishing, 1999
~ *The Miracle of Mindfulness.* Thich Nhat Hahn. Beacon Press, 1975, or the Classic Edition, Rider and Co., 2008
~ *Mindfulness In Plain English.* Bhante H. Gunaratana, Wisdom Publications, 2002
~ *10 Mindful Minutes: Giving Our Children—And Ourselves—the Social and Emotional Skills to Reduce Stress and Anxiety for Healthier, Happier Lives.* Goldie Hawn, with Gwen Holden. Perigee Books, 2011
~ *Just One Thing: Developing a Buddha Brain One Simple Practice at a Time.* Rick Hanson, Ph.D. New Harbinger Publications, Inc. 2011
~ *Energy Medicine for Women.* Donna Eden with David Feinstein, Ph.D. New York: Penguin Group, 2008
~ *Your Best Brain Ever:* National Geographic guide. Michael Sweeney, Ph.D., and Cyntha R. Green. Release date: Dec. 31, 2013
~ *Rewire Your Brain: Think Your Way to a Better Life.* John B. Arden, Ph.D. John Wiley and Sons, Inc., 2010
~ *Brain Gym: Simple Activities for Whole-Brain Learning.* Paul E. Dennison, Ph.D., and Gail E. Dennison. Edu-Kinesthetics, Inc, 1986
~ *Making a Good Brain Great.* Daniel Amen, M.D. Three Rivers Press, 2006
~ *The Brain Diet;* Alan C. Logan, N.D., FRSH; Cumberland House, 2006

~ *WHOLE: Rethinking the Science of Nutrition.* T. Colin Campbell, Ph.D., with Howard Jacobsen, Ph.D. Ben Bella Books, Inc., 2013
~ *Power Foods for the Brain,* Neal D. Barnard, M.D. Hachette Book Group, New York, 2013
~ *The Dark Side of Wheat.* Sayer Ji. e-book: http://www.greenmedinfo.com
~ *Grain Brain*: The Surprising Truth about Wheat, Carbs, and Sugar—Your Brain's Silent Killers. David Perlmutter, M.D. and Kristin Loberg, *Release Date:* September 17, 2013
~ *Green Smoothie Revolution: The Radical Leap Towards Natural Health.* Victoria Boutenko. North Atlantic Books, 2009

Articles:
~ *"A Workout for Your Brain, on Your Smartphone."* Kit Eaton. The New York Times, June 12, 2013
~ "Preventing Alzheimer's: Exercise Still Best Bet." Angela Lunde. *Mayo clinic.com,* 2008 http://www.mayoclinic.com/health/alzheimers/MY00002
~ *"Evolutionary Origins of Your Right and Left Brain."* Peter F. MacNeilage, Lesley J. Rogers, Giorgio Vallortigara. *Scientific American.* June 24, 2009
~ "Meditation as Medicine." Amy Paturel, MS. *Neurology Now,* August 2012
~ *"Reference Guide to Aerobic Exercise: An In-Depth Look",* by Jen Mueller and Nicole Nichols. http://www.sparkpeople.com/resources/fitness_articles
~ "Preventing Suicide." *Centers for Disease Control and Prevention,* September 10, 2012. http://www.cdc.gov/features/preventingsuicide/

Publications:
~ Strength training guide:
   http://www.cdc.gov/physicalactivity/growingstronger/
~ *Scientific American Mind,* http://www.scientificamerican.com/sciammind/
~ *Greater Good:* The Science of a Meaningful Life:
   http://www.greatergood.berkeley.edu/
~ *AARP Magazine:* http://www.aarp.org/magazine
~ *Mindful:* Taking Time for What Matters: http://www.mindful.org
~ *Experience Life* Magazine: http://www.experiencelife.com
~ *World's Healthiest Foods:* www.whfoods.org

Audiovisual:
~ *Utube has thousands* of free videos on brain health. You can bookmark or save some that you like. At http://www.utube.com in the search bar, type: "brain exercises" or "brain fitness" or "brain games" or "brain training", etc.
~ Free audio, video and slides: http://www.wisebrain.org
~ GreenMedTV: videos on health, nutrition, environment:
   http://tv.greenmedinfo.com/

~ Meditation: Free audio instruction. http://www.dhammatalks.org
~ Brain Sync sells recordings for memory, concentration, relaxation:
  http://www.brainsync.com

Community brain fitness centers
These are examples. There may be similar programs near you:
~ "Brainworks" program, Memorial Hospital of South Bend, Indiana:
  http://www.qualityoflife.org/memorialcms/index.cfm/brainworks/
~ Millenium Cognitive Café ^{SM} mobile brain training center:
  http://brainfitnessswfl.com/
~ Neurofeedback, Center for Brain Training: www.centerforbrain.com

Games and Training
~ *The Memory Practice*, a brain fitness website with FREE, fun exercises:
  http://www.thememorypractice.com
~ Free online brain games: http://www.braingle.com/
~ To find more, search online under "brain training games"
Brain Training Programs, such as *PositScience, Cognift*, and *Lumosity* have a few free exercises, and charge a membership fee for the rest. You can find these and many other brain fitness programs on the internet.
Computer program (one example):
~ *NeuroActive Program:* 4 CDs of games and exercises for Windows and Mac systems. Available at http://www.amazon.com

Funny-Bone Workouts
~ The Laugh Doctor, Cliff Kuhn, MD http://www.natural-humor-medicine.com
~ Laughter Yoga International, http://www.laughteryoga.org
~ American School of Laughter Yoga, http://laughteryogaamerica.com
~ World Laughter Tour, http://www.worldlaughtertour.com/

Websites:
~ Human Memory: http://www.human-memory.net/index.html
~ *The Human Brain* – educational website of the Franklin Institute.
  http://www.fi.edu/learn/brain/index.html
~ Aging Research, Brain Health Corner:
  http://www.agingresearch.org/section/topic/brainhealthcorner
~ "On the Brain" Dr. Michael Merzenich, http://merzenich.positscience.com/
~ *Longevity* at About.com: http://longevity.about.com
~ BrainPages—All Things Brain: http://www.brainpages.org
~ *"Exercise Prescription"*, free. Over 1400 exercises:
  http://www.exrx.net/index.html
~ The Best Brain Possible: http://www.thebestbrainpossible.com/

~ Brain Facts: current news, information: http://www.brainfacts.org/
~ Alzheimer's Association: http://www.alz.org
~ "Neurobics" http://www.keepyourbrainalive.com/exercise
~ *SharpBrains,* on brain science: http://www.sharpbrains.com
~ Wellspring Institute for Neuroscience and Contemplative Wisdom: http://www.wisebrain.org/wellspring-institute
~ Preserve Your Brain; weekly updates: http://www.preserveyourbrain.com
~ Traumatic Brain Injury site: http://www.brainline.org
~ Nutritional Medicine, Dr. Joel Fuhrman: http://www.drfuhrman.com/
~ GreenMedInfo, natural health research: http://www/greenmedinfo.com
~ *Yoga Journal.* http://www.yogajournal.com/
~ Tai Chi exercises and information: http://www.everyday-taichi.com/
~ Tai Chi instructors in U.S.: http://www.AmericanTaiChi.net
~ Interactive Metronome Program: http://www.interactivemetronome.com
~ Mindfulness inspired by Thich Nhat Hahn: http://plumvillage.org
~ Mindfulness Based Stress Reduction program: http://www.umassmed.edu/cfm/stress/
~ Insight Meditation Center, Barre, Massachusetts: http://www.insightmeditationcenter.org
~ Bhavana Society Forest Monastery and Retreat Center: http://www.bhavanasociety.org
~ MindUP™ program of mindfulness in schools http://thehawnfoundation.org/mindup/
~ The Energy Medicine Institute: http://www.energymed.org/
~ *EMDR (Eye Movement Desensitization, Reprocessing)* for trauma victims: http://www.emdria.org
~ *Emotional Freedom Technique* (tapping), Gwen Bonnell: http://www.tapintoheaven.com

NOTES

Introduction
1. Neurogenesis in the adult human hippocampus, *Nature Medicine Journal,* October 1998.
2. Robin Brey, M.D., "Use It Or Lose It." *Neurology Now,* March 2010, p.5
3. Eleanor A. Maguire, "Navigation-related structural change in the hippocampi of taxi drivers." *Proceedings of the National Academy of Sciences,* April 11, 2000, pp. 4398–4403
4. Carla Hannaford, Ph.D., *Smart Moves: Why Learning Is Not All In Your Head,* Great River Books, 2005, 1995, p.125
5. Daniel G. Amen, M.D., *Making a Good Brain Great: The Amen Clinic Program for Achieving and Sustaining Optimal Mental Performance,* (New York: Three Rivers Press, 2006), p.133

Chapter 1: Your Brain Circuits
1. Sandra Aamodt, Ph.D. and Sam Wang, Ph.D. Welcome to Your Brain: Why You Lose Your Car Keys but Never Forget How to Drive and Other Puzzles of Everyday Life, *Bloomsbury, USA, 2008, p.90*
2. S.J. Buell, and P.D. Coleman, "Dendritic growth in the aged human brain and failure of growth in senile dementia." *Science,* November 16, 1979; 206(4420):854-6.
3. Jess Blumberg, "Brain Gain." *Baltimore Magazine,* April 2008 Web: http://baltimoremagazine.net
4. "Integrated brain restoration after ischemic stroke--and other interventions for managing inflammation and enhancing brain plasticity." *Alternative Medicine Review,* March 2009
5. "Plasticity in cortical motor upper-limb representation following stroke and rehabilitation: two longitudinal multi-joint FMRI case-studies." *Brain Topography,* April 2012. 25(2):205-19
6. Daniel G. Amen, M.D., *Magnificent Mind At Any Age: Natural Ways to Unleash Your Brain's Maximum Potential,* Three Rivers Press, 2009, p.52
7. Paul E. Dennison, Ph.D., and Gail E. Dennison, *Brain Gym: Simple Activities for Whole-Brain Learning,* Edu-Kinesthetics, Inc, 1986, p.3
8. Peter F. MacNeilage, Lesley J. Rogers, and Giorgio Vallortigara. "Evolutionary Origins of Your Right and Left Brain." *Scientific American,* June 24, 2009
9. Aaron P. Nelson, Ph.D., with Susan Gilbert. *The Harvard Medical School Guide to Achieving Optimal Memory.* McGraw-Hill, 2005, pp.15-16
10. John Ratey, M.D., *SPARK: The Revolutionary New Science of Exercise and the Brain,* Little, Brown and Company, 2013, p.40

11. David Perlmutter M.D., *Power Up Your Brain.* Hay House, 2011, p.87
12. "Reasons Why Active Neurons And Brain Cells Are Better Cells." *Cognifit,* 2013, http://www.cognifit.com/science/didyou-know/neurons

Chapter 2: How the Exercises Work

1. Deepak Chopra, Quantum Healing, pp.49-50
2. John Ratey, M.D., *SPARK: The Revolutionary New Science of Exercise and the Brain*, Little, Brown and Company, 2013, p.56
3. Norman Doidge, M.D., *The Brain That Changes Itself*, Penguin Books, 2007, p.87
4. Carla Hannaford, Ph.D., *Smart Moves: Why Learning Is Not All In Your Head,* Great River Books, 2005, 1995, p.131
5. Ibid, p.125
6. Daniel G. Amen, M.D., *Making a Good Brain Great: The Amen Clinic Program for Achieving and Sustaining Optimal Mental Performance,* (New York: Three Rivers Press, 2006), p.133
7. Brain Gym website, http://www.braingym.com
8. Daniel G. Amen, M.D., *Making a Good Brain Great: The Amen Clinic Program for Achieving and Sustaining Optimal Mental Performance,* (New York: Three Rivers Press, 2006), p.131
9. Interactive Metronome website: http://www.interactivemetronome.com
10. Jorg Blech, *Healing Through Exercise*, Da Capo Press, 2009, p.111

Chapter 3: Using This Book

1. Carla Hannaford, Ph.D., *Smart Moves: Why Learning Is Not All In Your Head,* Great River Books, 2005, 1995, p.131
2. Ibid, p.131
3. Clifford Kuhn, M.D., "Depression." *Natural-Humor-Medicine.com* Web, 2009. http://www.natural-humor-medicine.com/depression.html?utm_source=REFERENCES_R7
4. Carla Hannaford, Ph.D., *Smart Moves: Why Learning Is Not All In Your Head,* Great River Books, 2005, 1995, p.133

Chapter 4: Sample Exercises

1. Goldie Hawn, *Ten Mindful Minutes*, Penguin Group (USA), Inc., p.110

Chapter 5: Exercise Sets

1. Carla Hannaford, Ph.D., *Smart Moves: Why Learning Is Not All In Your Head,* Great River Books, 2005, 1995, p.137
2. Donna Eden, with David Feinstein, Ph.D., *Energy Medicine for Women,* (New York, Penguin Group, 2008), p.67

3. Barbara Mallory, http://www.feelingfree.net, February 2006

4. Melinda Wenner, "Moving Your Eyes Improves Memory, Study Suggests." *LiveScience*, January 11, 2008

5. Claudia Cummins. "Prescriptions for Pranayama." Yoga Journal; Web: *http://www.yogajournal.com/practice/673*

6. "Standing Forward Bend" *Yoga Journal*; Web: http://www.yogajournal.com/practice/478

7. Paul E. Dennison, Ph.D., and Gail E. Dennison. *Brain Gym Teacher's Edition*. Edu-Kinesthetics, Inc, 2010, p.83

8. Carla Hannaford, Ph.D., *Smart Moves: Why Learning Is Not All In Your Head,* Great River Books, 2005, 1995, p.137

9. Cecilia Koester, M.Ed., "Have You Heard of Brain Gym®?" *Movement-Based Learning,* 2012. Web: www.movementbasedlearning.com

10. Michael James Hamilton, L.Ac., *AURICULAR: Ear Acupuncture Handbook,* 2002

11. Paul E. Dennison, Ph.D., and Gail E. Dennison. *Brain Gym Teacher's Edition*. Edu-Kinesthetics, Inc, 2010, p.66

12. Claudia Cummins, "Prescriptions for Pranayama." *Yoga Journal*; *http://www.yogajournal.com/practice/673*

13. Paul E. Dennison, Ph.D., and Gail E. Dennison. *Brain Gym Teacher's Edition*. Edu-Kinesthetics, Inc, 2010, p.68

14. Carla Hannaford, Ph.D., *Smart Moves: Why Learning Is Not All In Your Head*, Great River Books, 2005, 1995, p.134

15. Michael Reed Gach, *Acupressure's Potent Points*, Bantam Books, 1990, page 54

16. Gwenn Bonnell, *Tap Into Heaven*, Web: http://www.tapintoheaven.com

17. "Alternating cerebral hemispheric activity and the lateralization of autonomic nervous function." Human Neurobiology, 1983;2(1):39-43. Web: http://www.ncbi.nlm.nih.gov/pubmed/6874437

18. "Channel Cleaning Breath." *Yoga Journal,* Web: http://www.yogajournal.com/poses/2487

19. "EEG changes during forced alternate nostril breathing." *Int. Journal of Psychophysiology*, Oct;18(1):75-9. Web: http://www.ncbi.nlm.nih.gov/pubmed/7876041

Chapter 6: Exercise Summary

1. Donna Eden, with David Feinstein, Ph.D., *Energy Medicine for Women,* (New York, Penguin Group, 2008), page 67

2. Barbara Mallory, http://www.feelingfree.net, February 2006

3. Lee Berk, M.D., quoted in *American School of Laughter Yoga* (Web): http://www.laughteryogaamerica.com

4. Clifford Kuhn, M.D., "Depression". *Natural-Humor-Medicine.com* Web, 2009. http://www.natural-humor-medicine.com/depression.html?utm_source=REFERENCES_R7

5. Dr. Swami Karmananda Saraswati, "Mysteries of the Pineal." *Yoga Magazine,* 1979. Web: yogamag.net/archives/1979/cmar79/pineal.shtml

6. Melinda Wenner, "Moving Your Eyes Improves Memory, Study Suggests." *LiveScience,* January 11, 2008

7. Rita Milios. *Tools for Transformation.* Milios, 2007, 2011

8. Carla Hannaford, Ph.D., *Smart Moves: Why Learning Is Not All In Your Head,* Great River Books, 2005, 1995, p.137

9. Cappachione, Lucia. *The Power of Your Other Hand: A Course in Channeling the Wisdom of the Right Brain*, Career Press, 2001, p.162

10. Kim Ranegar, "Using your other hand benefits your brain." *Lake Michigan Shore,* June 2011. Web: http://www.nwitimes.com/niche/shore

11. Cappachione, Lucia. *The Power of Your Other Hand: A Course in Channeling the Wisdom of the Right Brain.* Career Press, 2001, p.160

12. Kim Ranegar. "Using your other hand benefits your brain." *Lake Michigan Shore,* June 2011. Web: http://www.nwitimes.com/niche/shore

13. Philamena lila Desi, "SaTaNaMa Meditation." *Healing;* Web: http://www.healing.about.com/b/2012/04/03/sa-ta-na-ma-meditation.html

14. Herbert Benson, M.D., *The Relaxation Response*, Web: http://www.relaxationresponse.org

15. Paul E. Dennison, Ph.D., and Gail E. Dennison. *Brain Gym 2010 Teacher's Edition.* Edu-Kinesthetics, Inc, 2010, p.83

16. Claudia Cummins. "Prescriptions for Pranayama." *Yoga Journal*: http://www.yogajournal.com/practice/673

17. "Alternating cerebral hemispheric activity and the lateralization of autonomic nervous function." *Human Neurobiology,* 1983;2(1):39-43. Web: http://www.ncbi.nlm.nih.gov/pubmed/6874437

18. "Channel Cleaning Breath." *Yoga Journal,* Web: http://www.yogajournal.com/poses/2487

19 . "EEG changes during forced alternate nostril breathing." *Int. Journal of Psychophysiology*, Oct;18(1):75-9. Web: http://www.ncbi.nlm.nih.gov/pubmed/7876041

20. Amy Paturel, M.S., M.P.H., "Meditation as Medicine," *Neurology Now,* August /Sept. 2012

21. Dennison, Paul E., and Gail E. Dennison. *Brain Gym® Teacher's Edition.* Edu-Kinesthetics, Inc., 2010, p.68

22. Carla Hannaford, Ph.D., *Smart Moves: Why Learning Is Not All In Your Head,* Great River Books, 2005, 1995, p.134

23. Michael Reed Gach. *Acupressure's Potent Points.* Bantam, 1990, p.54

24. Gwenn Bonnell, *Tap Into Heaven*, Web: http://www.tapintoheaven.com

25. Cecilia Koester, M.Ed. "Have You Heard of Brain Gym®?" *Movement-Based Learning,* 2012. Web: http://www.movementbasedlearning.com
26. Michael James Hamilton, L.Ac. *AURICULAR: Ear Acupuncture Handbook,* 2002
27. Dennison, Paul E., and Gail E. Dennison. *Brain Gym® Teacher's Edition.* Edu-Kinesthetics, Inc., 2010, p.66
28. "Standing Forward Bend," *Yoga Journal;* Web: http://www.yogajournal.com/poses/478

Chapter 7: Mindful Meditation

1. Goldie Hawn. *10 Mindful Minutes.* Perigee Books, 2011, p.10
2. "Brain Waves and Meditation." Science Daily. March 31, 2010 Web: http://www.sciencedaily.com/releases/2010/03/100319210631.htm
3. *Psychiatry Research: Neuroimaging.* Volume 191, Issue 1, January 2011, pp. 36-43
4. Yi-Yuan Tang, Qilin Lu, Ming Fan, Yihong Yang, and Michael I. Posner. "Mechanisms of white matter changes induced by meditation." *Proceedings of the National Academy of Sciences,* June 26, 2012 ISSN 0027-8424, 06/2012
5. David Perlmutter M.D., *Power Up Your Brain.* Hay House, Inc. 2011
6. Bhante H. Gunaratana, *Mindfulness In Plain English.* Wisdom Publications, 2002, p.70
7. Ibid., p.71
8. Stanley, E. A., Schaldach, J. M., Kiyonaga, A., & Jha, A. P. (2011). Mindfulness-based Mind Fitness Training: A Case Study of a High-Stress Predeployment Military Cohort. *Cognitive and Behavioral Practice.* 18(4):566-576.
9. MindUp Website: http://thehawnfoundation.org/mindup/

Chapter 8: Nutrition

1. Paul Bendheim, M.D. *The Brain Training Revolution: A Proven Workout for Healthy Brain Aging.* Sourcebooks, 2009, pp.57-59
2. "Vitamin B-6 (Pyridoxine)." *University of Maryland Medical Center. Web:* http://www.umm.edu/altmed/articles/vitamin-b6-000337.html
3. T. Colin Campbell, Ph.D., with Howard Jacobsen, Ph.D. *WHOLE: Rethinking the Science of Nutrition.* Ben Bella Books, Inc., 2013, p.7
4. T. Colin Campbell, Ph.D., *The China Study.* Ben Bella Books, Inc., 2010, pp. 348-349
5. Alan C. Logan, N.D., FRSH. *The Brain Diet: The Connection Between Nutrition, Mental Health, and Intelligence.* Cumberland House, 2006

6. Dr. Joey Shulman. "Top 5 Omega-3 Rich Foods." *The Christian Post*, December 14, 2005
http://www.christianpost.com/news/top-5-omega-3-rich-foods-11462/
7. Sayer Ji. "MCT Fats Found In Coconut Oil Boost Brain Function In Only One Dose." *GreenMedInfo.com.* April 4, 2013 Web:
http://www.greenmedinfo.com/blog/mct-fats-found-coconut-oil-boost-brain-function-only-one-dose
8. "Iowa State University News Release". *Journal of Clinical Nutrition*, August 2004; vol 80: pp. 396-403
9. A.V. Witte, et al. "Caloric Restriction Improves Memory in Elderly Humans." *Proceedings of the National Academy of Science*, January 27, 2009: 1255-60
10. David Perlmutter, M.D. *Power Up Your Brain.* Hay House, Inc. p.89-91
11. American Chemical Society. "Blueberry juice improves memory in older adults." *ScienceDaily*, January 21, 2010.
12. David Perlmutter M.D., *Power Up Your Brain.* Hay House, 2011, p.93
13. Michelle Turcotte, MS, RD. "Herbs For Brain Health." *Livestrong,* April 4, 2010 *Web:* http://www.livestrong.com/article/101807-herbs-brain-health
14. Gary Wenk, Ph.D., "Why Cinnamon Is Good for Your Aging Brain." *Psychology Today* online, June 4, 2013 Web:
http://www.psychologytoday.com/blog/your-brain-food/201306/why-cinnamon-is-good-your-aging-brain
15. "Intake of flavonoid-rich wine, tea, and chocolate by elderly men and women is associated with better cognitive test performance." J Nutr. 2009 Jan;139(1):120-7 *Source:* GreenMedInfo Summary *on Web:*
greenmedinfo.com/article/intake-flavonoid-rich-wine-tea-and-chocolate-elderly-men-and-women-associated-better
16. "Plasma antioxidants from chocolate." *Nature*, August 28, 2003; 424, 1013; *Web:*
http://www.nature.com/nature/journal/v424/n6952/full/4241013a.html
17. "The Sweet Truth About Cocoa Butter." *National Confectioner's Association* PDF;
Web: http://nca.files.cms-plus.com/Sweet_Truth_Cocoa_Butter_WEB.pdf
18 "Neuroprotective properties of resveratrol in different neurodegenerative disorders".*Biofactors,* 2010 Sep-Oct;36(5):370-6. doi: 10.1002/biof.118.
Web: http://www.ncbi.nlm.nih.gov/pubmed/20848560
19. "Tea Could Improve Memory, Study Shows." *Science Daily*, November 1, 2004, Web:
http://www.sciencedaily.com/releases/2004/10/041030144110.htm
20. "Study Shows Caffeine Linked to Avoidance of Alzheimer's Disease." *WUSF News*, University of South Florida, June 6, 2012; *Web:*
http://wusfnews.wusf.usf.edu/post/study-shows-caffeine-linked-avoidance-alzheimer-s-disease

21. David DiSalvo. "What Caffeine Really Does To Your Brain." *Forbes,* July 26, 2012
22. "Mayo Clinic Study Discovers Potential Link Between Celiac Disease and Cognitive Decline." *Science Daily,* October 12, 2006
23. David Perlmutter, M.D. Personal Interview; March 17, 2013
24. Victoria Boutenko. *Green Smoothie Revolution: The Radical Leap Towards Natural Health.* North Atlantic Books, 2009, p.18

Chapter 9: Brains Love Laughing!

1. Laughter Yoga International: http://laughteryoga.org/
2. Response to Repetitive Laughter Similar to Effect of Repetitive Exercise." *American Physiological Society* Press Release, April 23, 2010 http://www.the-aps.org/mm/hp/Audiences/Public-Press/For-the-Press/releases/10/12.html
3. Mobbs, D., Humor Modulates the Mesolimbic Reward Centers; *Neuron,* December 2003 http://www.cell.com/neuron/retrieve/pii/S0896627303007517
4. Cliff Kuhn, M.D., Depression, *Natural-Humor-Medicine.com.* *http://www.natural-humor-medicine.com/depression.html*
5. http://www.youtube.com/watch?v=JTYbGYSRRVg
6. http://teamcoco.com/video/sanjay-gupta-laughter
7. http://www.laughteryogaamerica.com/

Chapter 10: Remedy For Stress

1. Mark Schwartz, "Robert Sapolsky discusses physiological effects of stress." *Stanford Report,* March 7, 2007; http://news.stanford.edu/news/2007/march7/sapolskysr-030707.html
2. Relaxation Response website: http://www.relaxationresponse.org

Chapter 11: Making New Grooves

1. "Ink Wants To Form Neurons, And An Artful Scientist Obliges." *Discover Magazine,* April 30, 2012
2. M.C. Bushnell, et.al. "Cognitive and emotional control of pain and its disruption in chronic pain." *Nature Reviews, Neuroscience.* June 2013 http://www.ncbi.nlm.nih.gov/pubmed/23719569 Review: http://nccam.nih.gov/research/results/spotlight/062113
3. Daniel Amen, M.D. *Making a Good Brain Great.* Harmony Books, New York, 2005; p.8
4. "Preventing Suicide." *Centers for Disease Control and Prevention,* September 10, 2012; Web: http://www.cdc.gov/features/preventingsuicide/
5. Daniel Amen, M.D. Making a Good Brain Great. Harmony Books, New York, 2005; pp.13-15

6. Ibid.

7. Emmons, R.A., and McCullough, M.E. (2003) "Counting blessings versus burdens: Experimental studies of gratitude and subjective well-being in daily life. *Journal of Personality and Social Psychology, 84*, 377-389.

8. "Rapid effects of brief intensive cognitive-behavioral therapy on brain glucose metabolism in obsessive-compulsive disorder." S. Saxena, et al. Molecular Psychiatry, January 8, 2008

9. Robert Shapiro, "Finger Flash Therapy Catches On." CNN.com/health, February 15, 2000

10. Dawson Church, Ph.D., et al. "Psychological Symptom Change In Veterans After Six Sessions of Emotional Freedom Technique (EFT): An Observational Study. "Wholistic Healing Publications. January 2009; Web: http://www.stressproject.org/documents/marshall.pdf

Chapter 12: So Much More

1. Angela Lunde. "Preventing Alzheimer's: Exercise Still Best Bet." *Mayoclinic.com,* March 2008
Web: http://www.mayoclinic.com/health/alzheimers/MY00002

2. "Exercise training increases size of hippocampus and improves memory." *Proceedings of the National Academy of Sciences*, February 15, 2011

3. David Perlmutter M.D., *Power Up Your Brain.* Hay House, 2011, p.89

4. Pascale Michelon. Weight Training Boosts Brain Functions. *The Memory Practice*, April 26, 2012; Web: http://www.thememorypractice.com/?p=1309

5. Pascale Michelon, *Max Your Memory.* DK Publishing, New York, 2012

6. Norman Doidge, M.D., *The Brain That Changes Itself*, Penguin Books, 2007, pp.87-88

7. Richard Restak, M.D., and Scott Kim. *The Playful Brain: The Surprising Science of How Puzzles Improve Your Mind.* Riverhead Trade, 2011, p.3.

8. Neurobics website: http://keepyourbrainalive.com/exercise.html

9. Paul Gabrielson. Why Your Brain Loves That New Song. *Science,* April 11, 2013, Web: http://news.sciencemag.org/sciencenow/2013/04/why-your-brain-loves-that-new-so.html

10. Galina Mindlin, Don DuRousseau, Joseph Cardillo. Your Playlist Can Change Your Life. *Sourcebooks, 2012*

11. "Importance of Sleep." *Harvard* Women's Health Watch. January 2006; http://www.health.harvard.edu/press_releases/

12. Erika Cooper, personal interview, March 10, 2013

13. Hyperbaric oxygen in the treatment of patients with cerebral stroke, brain trauma, and neurologic disease. National Institutes of Health, PubMed. Adv Ther. 2005 Nov-Dec;22(6):659-78. Web: http://www.ncbi.nlm.nih.gov/pubmed/16510383

14. David Perlmutter, M.D. Personal Interview; March 17, 2013
15. "Aromatherapy." *University of Maryland* Medical Center. Web: http://umm.edu/health/medical/altmed/
16. "Ambient odors of orange and lavender reduce anxiety and improve mood in a dental office." *Journal of Physiology and Behavior,* Sept. 15, 2005. 86(1-2):92-5, *GreenMedInfo* Abstract. Web: http://www.greenmedinfo.com/article/ambient-odors-orange-and-lavender-reduce-anxiety-and-improve-mood-dental-office
17. Daniel G. Amen, M.D. *The Brain In Love: 12 Lessons To Enhance Your Love Life.* Three Rivers, Press, New York, 2007; p.5
18. Dr Eva Selhub. "Nature and the Brain: Mental Detox from Info-toxicity." *Alive.* Web: http://www.alive.com/articles/view/23809/nature_and_the_brain

Index of Exercises

Continued on Next Page . . .

Index, Continued

About The Author

Ann Marina is a Brain Fitness instructor, certified through the American Council on Exercise. She has taught Yoga for 30 years, and is registered through the International Yoga Alliance.

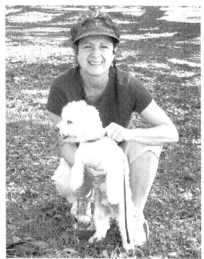

She also teaches Tai Chi and enjoys writing about natural health. Her work has appeared in *Family Magazine, Livestrong, Naples Daily News,* and on the *Alaska Public Radio Network.*

Ann was the founding publisher of *Alaskan Well-Being* magazine and resource directory in the 1980's.

She has led stress management and mind-body wellness courses at the University of Alaska and other learning centers.

She lives in Southwest Florida, where four-legged friend Dandy gets her out for brain-building fun.